Lesbian Studies: Setting An Agenda

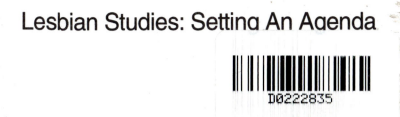

D0222835

Neither women's studies nor lesbian and gay studies have yet been able to offer an adequate theoretical or political framework for lesbians and lesbianism. Yet such a matrix is urgently needed, because the political and social position of lesbians is increasingly complex, especially in the light of the rise of the New Right and the new queer activism. *Lesbian Studies: Setting An Agenda* establishes such a matrix and provides an academic approach to both gender and the erotic, clarifying the damaging influence of heterosexism and examining lesbian treatment in sociology, feminism, psychology, social policy, cultural studies, film theory and history.

In addition to setting an agenda for lesbian studies, this book provides a wide resource and catalyst for anyone interested in gender and the erotic, including students and professionals in gender studies, sociology and cultural studies.

Tamsin Wilton is Senior Lecturer in Health Studies at the University of the West of England, Bristol.

Lesbian Studies:
Setting An Agenda

Tamsin Wilton

London and New York

First published 1995
by Routledge
11 New Fetter Lane, London EC4P 4EE

Simultaneously published in the USA and Canada
by Routledge
29 West 35th Street, New York, NY 10001

© 1995 Tamsin Wilton

Typeset in Times by LaserScript, Mitcham, Surrey
Printed and bound in Great Britain by
Mackays of Chatham PLC, Chatham, Kent

British Library Cataloguing in Publication Data
A catalogue record for this book is available from the British Library

Library of Congress Cataloguing in Publication Data
A catalogue record for this book has been requested

ISBN 0–415–08655–8 (hbk)
ISBN 0–415–08656–6 (pbk)

For all my lesbian friends, too many to name

Contents

Preface

Writing this has been both gruelling and exhilarating because of the subject matter and the circumstances in which it was written, and both are germane to the politics of the book. I am sure that many readers (and certainly those who are lone parents) will know exactly what I mean when I say that I had to squeeze it in between my 'proper' tasks. As I snatched precious hours at the keyboard in between cooking, cleaning, doing the shopping, feeding the cats, washing and ironing clothes, getting my son to school, to the dentist, to the homeopath, to the optician, looking after him when he was sick, watering the garden, paying the bills . . . oh, yes, and a full time university teaching job – my conviction that the personal is sure as hell political developed a new, sharp edge. When, in the middle of February and Chapter 4, I moved house, into a building site with no running water, no bathroom, no kitchen and no heating, my friends decided that this was the biggest and best displacement activity any writer could need.

This saga is told not to elicit sympathy (though any information leading to the location of a supermarket which delivers will be duly rewarded!), nor to excuse the shortcomings of the text, but to hammer home the point that lesbians – after all the theoretical deconstructing which goes on in these pages – *are*, in the material here and now, *women*. That is one reason why 'lesbian and gay studies' is *not* an adequate arena within which to theorise lesbian-ness,[1] just as women's studies is not. Only by working within a specific arena dedicated to and named as 'lesbian studies' can we map a feminist critique of the power relations inherent in what Gayle Rubin calls the sex/gender system on to the exhilarating gender-fuck of queer politics (and vice versa).

That my subject matter proved gruelling will also come as no surprise to many readers. When I teach or write about the oppression of lesbians – the silencing and distortion of lesbian voices, the mutilation of lesbian bodies, the cruel penalties suffered by women throughout history for desiring and pleasuring each other, the breaking of lesbian hearts – I am writing about my people. The flip side of this is exhilaration. When I teach or write about who lesbians are or have been – the wit of Woolf's *Orlando*, the defiant stylishness of Gluck, the fury of Lavendar Menace, the awesome courage of Audre Lorde, the intellectual audacity of Monique Wittig, the erotic lyricism of Suniti Namjoshi and Gillian Hanscombe, the warmth and integrity of Joan Nestle . . . and this list could go on for pages – I am also writing about my people. And in this act of writing I claim a people for myself, I make myself lesbian.

On this level, as on the level of material inequality, deconstructing 'lesbian' simply doesn't matter. Of course it makes no sense at all to ask, 'Was Sappho a lesbian?' because it is the wrong question (see pp. 53–5). But that revered profile on ancient coinage belongs to the woman for whom I was named 'sapphic', 'lesbian'. That makes her and me now one people. And it is this heady and unmanageable brew of academic rigour and self-conscious myth-making, of material analysis and post modern game-playing, that makes Lesbian Studies what it is.

So much for the 'lesbian'. What about the 'studies'? As the first member of my working-class, Cornish family to go to university, I am made deeply uneasy by those feminists who reject the academic enterprise as inherently patriarchal. To me that makes about as much sense as saying that women shouldn't learn how to fix cars because technology is inherently patriarchal. *Nothing* is inherently masculine/feminine or inherently patriarchal. Many of our most important lesbian writers and activists work in the academy and do so, presumably, because they think it matters. To me, it matters enormously. The academy is a place of transformation, of incitement to learning (Lorde 1984), of disobedience. Yes, it is here and now a heteropatriarchal[2] institution, but that makes it special? We need lesbians *everywhere*.

Students in my women's studies classes often complain that theoretical language is exclusive and inaccessible. They often add for good measure that in consequence it is classist and racist. This is a charge which continues to crop up from time to time in feminist circles, though I am not aware that students of medicine, mechanical engineering or particle physics feel the same. And that is the point. If you want to learn about quarks and Buckminsterfullerenes, torsion or mitochondria, you expect to learn a specialist language. What is more, as Anne Eisenberg reminds us, 'to be safe, one must regard technical language as a language apart from ordinary speech' (Eisenberg 1991). The complexities of gender and of sexuality, especially in their mutual inflections, are no less awesome than those of wave/particle duality. The politics comes in what *use* you make of specialist language. When you use jargon and mystification to prop up your self-esteem and to establish a hierarchy with you at the top and anyone who can't understand what you are saying at the bottom, that is oppressive.

The academy is rife with oppressive practices because it is not just about learning, it is about gate-keeping and reputations, jumping through hoops and collecting letters after your name, all of which have in time-honoured style been used to exclude people of the wrong colour, gender, class, age or dis/ability. But you can refuse to play those games. You can demystify jargon, widen access to and understanding of specialist language, so that theory becomes a tool for anyone who wants to use it rather than the foundational property of the elite. As women, we are *supposed* to be illogical and unintelligent, we are *supposed* not to be able to understand complex language, so that refusing to engage with theory at any but the most basic level colludes with our own oppression. None of which means that it is either possible or desirable to write the *Ladybird Book of Lesbian Feminist Theory*.

My class background, my gender, my whiteness, my sexuality and my commitment to teaching and learning have informed the writing of this book, as the various positions of its readers will inform different meanings for it. It deals with theory, with activism and with the material circumstances of lesbian lives. It is academic, but it is certainly not 'detached'. The lesbian brings with her into the academy[3] her unruly lesbian body, her desire, lust, love, stigma, her voice, anger, fear and disobedience. These are all things which I believe the academy could well do with. For me, becoming a lesbian was like lighting the blue touch paper beneath a firework. I believe that a similar re-energising is possible for the academy. From a lesbian perspective, the heterosexist academy seems intellectually stagnant, weighed down by anachronism and unable to perceive the ideological imperative which hampers it. That is why a lesbian perspective is what the academy so desperately needs, and it is why I found the space to write this book.

Bristol, November 1994

NOTES

1   Throughout this book I will refer to 'lesbian-ness' rather than 'lesbianism'. The latter carries overtones of pathology (astigmatism, aneurism, lesbianism) which I reject. It is also too specific – I feel uneasy writing about the 'lesbianism of a text', for example – while lesbian-ness, like richness or loveliness, holds a more flexible set of meanings.

2 I follow the practice of referring to 'heteropatriarchy' rather than simply 'patriarchy' in order to foreground the co-dependency of sexism and heterosexism in the maintenance of male supremacy. The subordination of women within/by the regime of gender is inseparable from the oppression and abjectification of lesbians and gay men.

3 She also brings all these things into the supermarket, the synagogue, the mosque, the factory, the sauna . . . wherever she goes. The academy is just one more place for a dyke to go.

Acknowledgements

By its very nature, this book is the fruit of many people's labour, although its shortcomings are entirely my responsibility. I owe a great debt to everyone whose work I have made use of here, especially early pioneers in this field such as Margaret Cruikshank, whose courage in writing about lesbian-ness must have been quite extraordinary. In the same vein I would like to thank Ken Plummer, Joseph Bristow and Jeffrey Weeks, whose hard work on behalf of lesbian and gay studies has made it possible for me and many others to make contact with other lesbian and gay scholars in Britain. Thanks, too, to Diane Richardson, Sue Wilkinson, Lisa Adkins, Norma Daykin, Helen (charles), Jackie Stacey and Celia Kitzinger, whose readiness to engage in discussion has been so stimulating. Many ideas are tempered during the course of my teaching, and I must record my gratitude to the students on my 'Feminist Approaches to Sexuality' option during 1993, who were so ruthless in not letting me get away with waffle! I am indebted to my colleague Lesley Doyal, whose experienced – and always tactful – guidance in honing my writing skills has been invaluable. Thanks are due to the anonymous reader at Routledge, whose thoughtful comments on the original proposal resulted in a much stronger (and longer) book, to Gill Davis for her initial enthusiasm, to Elizabeth Tribe for her encouragement and support, and to Heather Gibson for her patience. Finally, I would not have been able to write a word without the affectionate tea-making skills of my son, Tom Coveney, or the support of my lesbian friends in Bristol.

Introduction
Lesbian *what*?

'If it were not lesbian, this text would make no sense'

(Brossard 1985)

This is 'the Golden Age of gay and lesbian studies' (Plummer 1992: 3) and, as such, there could be no better time to begin carving out space for lesbian studies. Lesbian and gay studies is an innovative and rapidly expanding academic enterprise. It was founded on the theoretical interventions of lesbian feminism, which itself developed from inadequacies in heterosexual feminism and women's studies, and which shifted lesbian and gay intervention outwards from the homophile activism of the 1950s and 1960s towards a more rigorous and proactive challenge to heterosexual hegemony.

Lesbian studies has always occupied a precarious position on the cusp of women's studies and lesbian and gay studies/queer studies. Marginalised by and within both, the social phenomenon of lesbian invisibility has been compounded. From the perspective of gay and lesbian studies, Plummer suggests: 'There has been the classic split between lesbians and gays, whereby many lesbians find their interests better served by the more fully developed women's studies while gay men remain largely aloof, patronizing, naive or simply threatened' (ibid.: 10). While it is true that women's studies is 'more fully developed' as an academic presence, it has been too saturated with homophobia to develop a radical critique of the erotic, or to offer an intellectually adequate milieu for lesbians. As Katie King comments, 'Lesbian theory, fiction, scholarship, activist writing, once occupying a center (if not the center) of feminist "thought", has now been displaced in the academy' (King 1990: 88).

The purpose of this book is to establish tentative pathways through and towards a body of enquiry which may be called with some confidence lesbian studies. One theme which may be traced throughout is the inadequacy of both feminism and queer theory as sites for lesbian speech, and the insights which lesbian studies may have to offer both. Another major theme is the intellectual naivety of traditional academic disciplines. Within many disciples (such as social policy) the possibility of lesbian existence goes unrecognised; within some (such as psychology) it is pathologised; within others it is rendered impossible within/by the dominant paradigm of inquiry (this is true of film studies, for example, whose dominant paradigm is monolithically heterosexual). Thus, the academic apparatus appears to the lesbian scholar not as the neutral, value-free pursuit of something called 'truth' or 'knowledge', which is how it presents itself, but as an inherently ideological enterprise obedient to and supporting an intellectually numbing heterobinarism.[1] Lesbian studies is, then, inherently an agent of the postmodern fragmentation of the rationalist project, and one of our tasks becomes to identify and speak from a specifically *lesbian* truth-position within and about every scholarly discipline.

Leakage across disciplinary boundaries is entirely appropriate to lesbian studies. For as 'lesbian' is constructed within and by a multitude of discourses, so lesbian studies must be mapped on to and across a broad field, ignoring or fracturing traditional disciplinary boundaries and turning the insights of one on to the praxis of another. It will, however, probably infuriate the specialist reader, as will the inevitably incomplete representation of each specialism touched on in these few pages.

There are many important absences here, absences which I regret but which are inevitable if this book is to be small enough for you to hold in your hand. I have not been able to discuss lesbian spirituality for example (see Butler (ed.) 1990, Curb and Manahan 1985, Stuart 1992), nor what a lesbian presence in the 'hard' sciences might consist of, nor important issues around lesbian cultural activism, including lesbian intervention in the politics of HIV/AIDS (see Leonard 1990, Patton 1985, Schneider 1992). I have not had space to discuss the presence of lesbians on network television, nor lesbian video,[2] including the British queer video magazine *Pout*. I particularly regret not having enough space to address lesbian philosophy (see Card (ed) 1992, Lucia-Hoagland 1988). Such gaps, sadly, are unavoidable, and I hope others will write them into the lesbian studies programme.

LESBIAN CONTENT, LESBIAN PRAXIS

The book opens with an attempt to define and situate lesbian studies, discussing its relationship to queer studies and to women's studies, and its general position in the academy at this point in time. Any attempt to stake out intellectual territory for lesbian studies must engage with the problematic nature of a liberatory politics predicated upon its status as stigmatised 'other' within the discursive regime of heteropatriachy. By refusing the ideological imperative by which we are defined and cast out of the body politic, by deconstructing 'lesbian' as a disciplinary sign instrumental in the social control of women and of sexuality, we render the subject and object of lesbian studies both archaic and politically contaminated. This is not unique to lesbian studies. Gay studies is obliged to recognise that 'a true liberation would also dissolve the very object of liberation, the homosexual, since the idea itself is predicated upon the very distinctions to be attacked' (Plummer 1992: 7), while feminism must answer the question, 'If "woman" is merely a social construct, then what price women's liberation?' (Wilton 1992: 74). Establishing a field of study around the existence of a group whose identity *as* a group is a response to their oppression is a charged and problematic project.

The next problem implicit in the attempt to define lesbian studies is the equally thorny question of lesbian identity itself. Ransacking the 'lesbians' constructed in a range of phallocentric/androcentric discourses, variously positioned relative to gender, the erotic, the pathological and the political, a semantic question is swiftly revealed as a strategic and political one – a kind of paradigmatic twitch which will become more and more familiar during the course of the book's argument. Faced with a protean shape-shifter 'lesbian', so multiform as to become, ironically, slippery and invisible, the naming of lesbians begins to seem a curious matter indeed. Elizabeth Grosz says of feminism, 'feminist theory should consider itself a form of *strategy*. Strategy involves recognizing the situation and alignments of power within and against which it operates' (Grosz 1990a: 59). This is true for lesbian studies. A naming-of-lesbian based in a radical critique of heteropatriarchal 'alignments of power' is strategically necessary in the struggle against lesbian oppression and in the establishment of anti-heteropatriarchal readings and a queer–feminist academic praxis.

This radical naming-as-lesbian becomes immediately problematic when we turn to the subject of the next chapter, history. Lesbians have been subject to erasure from the record, of that there can be no doubt. It is not possible, however, to write them back in, in any straightforward way. Sexual identity is a reflexive self-narrative profoundly dependent on cultural, economic and social factors – such as the availability of the notion of 'sex' or 'identity' – all of which are subject to quite dramatic shifts, sometimes over remarkably short intervals. Scrutinising social history makes clear the contingent and constructed nature of all sexualities. Essentialist models of sexuality simply disintegrate when we attempt to map them on to the Macedonia of Philip and Alexander, the Americas of the First Peoples, the England of Marlowe or Katherine Philips. If it makes no sense to call Sappho a lesbian it means little enough to use the word to name as recent a figure as Radclyffe Hall, so different was its meaning in her life. So, although I join in the process of writing lesbians into the historical record, it is with a cautious awareness of the partial and flawed nature of that undertaking and an insistence on the greater importance of understanding the ebb and flow of meaning which adheres to *our* word 'lesbian' when we make use of it to catalyse a particular reading of history.

From the beginnings of the modern period, sexual behaviours have been subject to something of a taxonomic onslaught, and it is this which is the focus of the next chapter. Insisting that the various models of sexual identity, whatever the contradictions among and within them, are neither defunct nor harmless, this chapter critiques several key candidates. Against a background detailing the recent history of competing truth claims concerning (homo)sexuality, Freudian psychoanalytical and biomedical models are examined in as much depth as space allows, and the outlines of the essentialism/constructionism debate are sketched in. I take as given the political nature of attempts to categorise sexuality, and my aim in this chapter is to develop a strategic response which exposes and engages with the major models of sexual identity *as* political texts. Furthermore, the *gendering* of sexualities, which is such an inextricable feature of most taxonomies of the erotic, has interesting and important consequences. Questions of phallocentricity, and of lesbian sexual agency as either obedient or disobedient to the symbolic hegemony of the phallus, are live and unresolved in lesbian feminism and in lesbian cultural and political praxis.

'Lesbian feminism' is not in itself a straightforward notion, including as it does a history of mutual antagonism as well as a pungent set of disagreements among lesbians concerning the relationship – if any – between lesbian-ness and feminism. Chapter 5 narrates the troubled history of the lesbian presence within the women's liberation movement and attempts to theorise the so-called 'gay/straight split' which so many commentators have described within second-wave feminism. I find it quite extraordinary that feminism has become for so many commentators some kind of restrictive mother, a powerful and repressive orthodoxy, when in fact the position of feminism remains both tentative and vulner-able. I also find it disturbing that feminism is rejected as erotophobic by vocal sections of the lesbian community, and one of my aims here is to explore this set of contradictions further.

I tend to agree with Katie King that 'inside feminism, the term gay/straight split marks a kind of mistake: the assumption that differ-ences among women are only bipolar. Instead, differences come to be seen as simultaneously creating and created, strategically positioned' (King 1990: 83). Yet there *is* substance of some kind to the continuing refusal of non-lesbian feminism to incorporate a lesbian perspective, or to deal respectfully with lesbians, and I suggest that this rests upon two questions. One is male violence, the other the failure of feminism to move beyond the deconstruction of gender and the problem of sexual difference. At the heart of these two issues lie the antagonism which non-lesbian feminism clearly expresses towards lesbian feminists and the bitterness of the division among lesbians between sex-radicals and revolutionary feminists. I propose that a solution to the current political impasse in feminism may be found in a radical interpenetration of feminist with queer theory, taking Judith Butler's demand that we 'trouble gender' as a starting point.

If truth-telling is understood as only a privileged kind of story-telling, then stories themselves may be seen in a different light. As with any oppressed group, telling a *lesbian* story has taken on an importance outwith purely aesthetic considerations. The chapter on lesbian literary studies explores both that importance and the uses of lesbian reading in constructing lesbian subjectivity and in making a place for 'lesbian' outwith the heteropatriarchal master-narrative. The processes of writing and reading as a lesbian, the location of lesbian-ness in literary texts, the difficulties of teaching lesbian literature – all have been widely debated (see Hobby and White (eds) 1991, Jay and Glasgow (eds) 1992, Munt 1992, Zimmerman 1992a). Less theorised are the implications of lesbian readings and lesbian texts for traditional literary scholarship, where we may position questions of sexuality in relation to the canon (see Sedgwick 1990) and where we may situate lesbian-ness within feminist lit crit. Since there has been a veritable explosion of lesbian fiction and poetry published in recent years, with concomitant developments in lesbian literary theory, this chapter suffers perhaps more than any other in the book from trying to cram complex debates and a vast body of work into a few pages.

Cultural studies has been the site of diverse interventions from groups whose position is eccentric to the mainstream. The position of lesbian-ness among this polyvocality is an intriguing one and deserves at least a book of its own. This chapter focuses on the visual and time-based media and, in particular, on painting, film and music. This is partly motivated by pragmatism: there is more written about painting and film in feminist and queer theory than about dance, theatre or music. It would, however, be strange indeed to ignore music, which is apparently such a lively and central presence in lesbian social life, and I have made the tentative beginnings of a lesbian exploration of music.

The book concludes with a discussion of lesbian-ness from a sociological perspective and with an analysis of the lesbian in relation to social policy. Sociology has been one of the first disciplines to develop a specifically lesbian and gay practice, and it was within sociology that the germ of constructionism first took root with the publication of Mary McIntosh's article 'The homosexual role' (McIntosh 1968). Traditionally regarded as a political radical within the academy, sociology has much to offer lesbian studies. Indeed, much early lesbian writing may be located within sociology, as women described, analysed and theorised the social position of lesbians (for example, Abbott and Love 1972, Darty and Potter 1984, Klaich 1985). This informal sociology, which includes autobiographical and oral-historical accounts, is a genre which continues to hold a central place in grass-roots lesbian scholarship as well as within the academy. Here, feminist epistemological and methodological developments are of key importance for the development of a radical pro-lesbian sociological praxis.

The role of women as unpaid carers is central to capitalism, whether in the British Welfare State (being dismantled, as I write, by the longest-lived right-wing administration this century) or in the free market. Lesbians, although especially vulnerable under policy regimes which do not recognise our existence, are not exempt from this caring obligation: many care for children, for elderly and infirm parents or for partners. Nor are lesbians able to escape from the economic penalties consequent on being female in a state dependent on a heterosexual division of labour. The final chapter outlines the problems faced by lesbian citizens – problems related to both gender and sexuality – and points to the implications for a (so far inadequate) feminist critique of social policy.

MOVING FORWARD

Any lesbian studies which neglected the feminist critique of the power relations of gender would be a feeble creature indeed. Yet queer theory, for all its political narrowness, offers strategic interventions in the field of gender which mainstream feminism does not. Queer, too, has much to offer lesbian studies. Yet lesbian studies is much more than a straight-forward blend of queer and feminism. Ironically, both feminism and queer, albeit from very different positions, may be said to constitute reinscriptions of phallocentricity, and hence replicate that which they seek to displace. To the extent that 'lesbian' is the *only* position utterly outwith the regime of Irigary's *hommosexual* exchange, and to the extent that it is also the only sign which refuses to attach itself to the phallus (although it may play with it), lesbian studies may offer a site for profoundly radical revisioning and a fundamentally disobedient intel-lectual praxis.

Simply enacting lesbian agency places us outside heteropolarity, although, as lesbian writers frequently warn, the rupture of 'lesbian' from hetero-relations must not be assumed. Indeed, some (Meese 1992, Traub 1991) assert that such a rupture is impossible. While it seems to me *not* impossible, only a continuing reflexivity, an endless process of renegotiation, repositioning and recoding 'lesbian' can effect our resist-ance to recuperation.

> The illusionary and visionary project (it must be both of these) of lesbianism is to be writing the 'beyond' of heterosexual phallo-gocentrism, even though this is what is always recuperating us, claiming to (re)produce us as one of its effects.
>
> (Meese 1992: 82)

'Lesbian', then, is indeed a privileged signifier, a magical sign. Or, rather, lesbian-ness is a privileged site of inquiry. For I agree with Marilyn Farwell that 'lesbian' must be seen as a *position*, not a type of person, if lesbian theory is to move beyond the epistemological and symbolic limits of heterobinarism. 'Ahistoricism and essentialism', Farwell writes, 'are the central problems which have plagued the attempt to define lesbian metaphorically. I believe that some of those problems are eliminated when one speaks of lesbian as a space rather than as an essence' (Farwell 1992: 102).

This approach offers an important strategy for pre-empting ghetto-isation and intellectual marginalisation. Lesbian studies, if it is to be of anything other than curiosity value – and certainly if it is to affect the radical shifts across the academy which I propose in this book – must be accessible to non-lesbians. 'Lesbian' as a space, a position, is of course open to general occupation. And it is in this that lesbian studies offers the most fundamental revisioning of feminism. Reading texts *with a lesbian eye* is the *only* strategy whereby feminism may develop a critique of heterosexuality as an institution and of the co-dependency of gender and the erotic in constructing and maintaining heteropatriarchal relations of power. It also offers a way out of the impasse in which women's studies currently finds itself, trapped in the multiple sets of inherited power relations deployed along axes of difference. Katie King refers to:

> [A] division of labour which is sometimes characterized as the 'theory' of white women built on the 'experiences' of women of colour; or in a move that keeps these ranges appropriately separated – the 'theory' of heterosexual academics, built on the 'experiences' of lesbians.
>
> (King 1990: 89)

This highlights the central problem of lesbian studies. For 'lesbian' carries something akin to the paradox of wave/particle duality, being at one and the same time a theoretical construct and a living woman who is materially endangered. The notion of 'lesbian-as-space' is, I suspect, the only way out of that paradox. For, if 'lesbian' is a space then, rather than exploiting lesbian labour and lesbian oppression in the service of a 'general' (read 'heterosexual') feminist theory, heterosexual academics may take responsibility for speaking from that space, may do lesbian labour themselves. I do not have any naive optimism about this – it requires that non-lesbian feminists critique their own heterosexual privilege, and this is a demand which has met demonstrably with stubborn resistance (see, for example, Wilkinson and Kitzinger (eds) 1993). Yet the essays in this book assume that it is only by making the position 'lesbian' available to the whole range of differently gendered, sexed and desiring subjects that the apparatus of lesbian oppression may be dismantled and the limits of the academic enterprise transcended. The radical question for and of lesbian studies is, in the words of Elizabeth Meese:

> What path can lead us to the 'yes' of 'the lesbian' beyond the male–female opposition of hetero-relational feminism . . . 'the lesbian' beyond the Derridean refusal of lesbianism as homosexuality's opposition to heterosexuality?
>
> (Meese 1992: 83)

It is this central question which this book, skimming as it does over a handful of academic disciplines, poses. And, in posing it, it must be remembered that 'None of this is easy. It requires an effort in mind for which there are no certain signs' (ibid.: 83). What follows, then, is a set of uncertain signs, mapping out a space 'lesbian' and a powerfully chaotic agenda for lesbian studies.

NOTES

1 I use 'heterobinarism' to refer to the way in which a binary model posited on the supposed complementarity of two sexes has become conceptually dominant in Western thinking. Everything from electrical engineering (male plugs and female sockets) to art crit. (where a brush stroke may be 'virile' or 'feminine') is saturated with the language of heterosex as constructed within patriarchal power relations.

2 This is an important omission, since lesbian video is increasingly important to lesbian culture. Not only are lesbian porn and safe sex videos contributing to a *lesbian* construction of lesbian sex, but important independent lesbian film is often distributed on video. See, for example, *Lesbian Lykra Shorts*, which includes films by four lesbian film-makers and which is distributed by Dangerous to Know (UK telephone no.: 0171 735 8330).

Chapter 1

Deviant pedagogies
The nature of lesbian studies

To propose lesbian studies as an academic discipline is to open the floodgates to a deluge of doubts, queries and contradictions. What is the purpose of lesbian studies, who is it for and what are its disciplinary and pedagogic boundaries? Does the name 'lesbian studies' refer to scholarship in any field undertaken *by* lesbians, or to the study *of* lesbians and lesbian issues? Should students and/or teachers be lesbians? Whose interests should we prioritise, why and how? What place is there in lesbian studies for political struggles against lesbian oppression within and by the academy? What is the relationship of lesbian studies to the academy; a new subject area struggling for validation and acceptance, or a praxis intended to disrupt utterly and subvert the structures and assumptions of the academy itself? Is it possible for a distinct and autonomous area of scholarship to be predicated upon the existence within contemporary societies of a deviant and stigmatised sexual minority, a minority moreover whose very nature shifts fundamentally among temporal and geographical locations?

Such questions are familiar to women's studies (see Bowles and Duelli Klein (eds) 1983, Brimstone 1991, Rich 1981b). Questions of identity – of who studies whom – seem to parallel the dilemma for women of how far and in what way they should co-operate with men. This question has long proved problematic in the context of women's studies (Mahony 1983), and is further complicated for lesbian studies by the unique relationship between lesbians and gay men. Another debate which has a familiar resonance is that concerning the contested position of lesbian studies *vis-à-vis* queer studies/sexuality studies/women's studies. How may we best engage in and with lesbian studies as a scholarly enterprise?

Until relatively recently, the nature of specific academic disciplines was not a matter of debate. Geography, history, modern languages, physics, mathematics, etc., had clearly recognised (if sometimes over-lapping) boundaries. Furthermore, the 'ivory tower' of academe was a space set apart, rising transcendentally above mundane concerns such as politics. But this is in itself a political position. Its privileges were founded on exclusivity and on its self-proclaimed characteristics of neutrality and objectivity. Members of marginalised groups were ex-cluded from the academy precisely because they were said to be incapable of such detached objectivity, either by nature or by reason of their vested interests in transformation. Being so excluded, their construction as ignorant and illogical was reinforced and their wider social disenfran-chisement compounded.

It was feminists who first pointed out that the academy was androcentric, that 'objectivity' was no more than a code word for the dominant male point of view, and that the 'truth' supposedly unearthed by male research was nothing more than men's *construction* of reality, deployed to further the interests of men as a class.[1] Black feminists added that the process and the product of the academy operated to perpetuate white ruling-class supremacy (Collins 1990, hooks 1990, Lorde 1982). Once revealed as being constructed around and repro-ducing an agenda which was both androcentric and ethnocentric, the ideological and political nature of academic 'objectivity' was exposed, and the way was opened for the theoretical legitimation of a range of alternative, oppositional pedagogies. Women's studies, black studies and, more recently, lesbian and gay studies and disability studies have made their way, not without struggle, on to higher education curricula in the USA and Europe.

Opposition to lesbian and gay studies has been fierce. Homophobia is the most respectable of prejudices, and it remains a majority view-point that a set of execrated, criminalised sexual practices is an inadequate foundation for an academic discipline. The vulnerable position of the academy itself serves to exacerbate hostility to what is clearly a politically risky enterprise in the climate of homophobia fostered by the ascendancy of fundamentalisms and fuelled by the Right's cynical appropriation of the AIDS crisis (Wilton 1992a). Ken Plummer, who has been instrumental in building an institutional foundation for lesbian and gay studies in Britain, outlines the problems:

> [A] press waiting to pounce, a university administration too scared to champion such work, students worried about careers and tenure,

colleagues who are homophobically entrenched. In the midst of all this controversy it is surprising that a lesbian and gay studies has come to exist at all.

(Plummer 1992: 11)

Yet exist it does. More established in the USA, with a broader academic network and firmer structural footing, it is growing at a phenomenal rate even in the doggedly insular milieu of Britain. This is not as new an enterprise as we might think. Since the earliest days of the homophile movement in the USA, groups such as the Daughters of Bilitis were beginning to explore lesbian-ness in a theoretical way as part of their integrationist endeavours, while an alternative university, the Institute for Homophile Studies, 'enrolled over 1,000 students in the academic year 1957–8' (Plummer 1992: 7). The Third Reich succeeded in wiping out not only a flourishing lesbian and gay subculture but a burgeoning academic infrastructure for sexuality studies that had sprung up in Germany after the First World War.

Infiltrating the academy, however, is not universally perceived as a Good Thing by groups traditionally excluded. Having recognised the limited and exclusive nature of traditional academic practice, such groups may decide that reforming the institution and its practices is an important political goal. On the other hand, they may simply argue that energy put into reform is energy wasted, that the risks of co-option and incorporation are too great. One alternative is a separatist strategy, establishing alternative institutions and practices, thereby resisting incorporation and, by the proliferation of oppositional practices and pedagogies, displacing the hetero-academy from its central, legitimate position. This debate has been a live one in women's studies, where it gains additional significance from the wider debate around separatism in general (Aaron and Walby 1991, Hawthorne 1991, Lowe and Lowe Benston 1991, Sheridan 1991).

It is not only by exclusion that the hetero-academy acts as the agent of various oppressions. It also constructs and legitimates a specific and limited set of discursive and pedagogic practices as the *only* true and authentic world view. The common-sense reality which most people experience themselves as 'inhabiting' is largely constructed within and by the operation of this narrow but extremely powerful world view. Any group whose social stigmatisation or marginalisation is mandated or legitimated by traditional academic discourse must both challenge or render illegitimate the discursive structuration which reflects and repro-duces its subordination and produce resistant/oppositional texts about the world and itself. In order for either strategy to be effective, however, it must itself be legitimate within the terms of engagement. Polemic may answer polemic but cannot pose an effective challenge to that which pretends to be objectively verifiable truth. The problem then becomes, to what extent should those seeking to challenge the academy do so on the academy's own terms, or to what extent expose the illegitimacy of academic discourse *per se*? For feminists, for example, the question becomes whether to reject theory *itself* as intrinsically masculine, or to construct theory which is feminist, oppositional and subversive of patriarchal practice (Douglas 1990).

LESBIAN/FEMINIST? FEMALE HOMOSEXUAL?

An additional complication is that power and powerlessness in our society are generally thought of in terms of a set of simple binary axes, such that Black is oppressed by white, female by male, homosexual by heterosexual, and so forth (Wilton 1992a). In fact, none of us exists in only one such group – it is, for example, impossible to be black and not be simultaneously gendered – and the structuring dynamics of any power differential between two individuals is seldom straightforward. Race, gender and sexuality infect and inflect one another in ways which have yet been barely recognised (Davis 1982, Fung 1991, Mercer 1991). The interests of those fighting different oppressions may be experienced as contradictory and/or conflicting.

It is precisely this conflicting nature of specific oppressions which makes the social, political and academic positioning of 'lesbian' so difficult. Lesbians are, by definition, women (though see below pp. 29–49), but we are also by definition homosexual. Then, too, although lesbian-ness plays a crucial role in radical feminist theory and politics, to be a lesbian is not a *necessarily* feminist position. For every radical lesbian feminist whose choice to love women springs from, or is at least informed by, a political identification with women, there is a non-feminist lesbian whose relation to women is experienced as primarily erotic, and who may with some justification perceive feminism as eroto-phobic and heterosexist. While some feminist lesbians may advocate political separatism from men, other lesbians may endorse wholeheart-edly the multiply gendered politics of Queer Nation. What are the implications of this for lesbians? Is it possible to reconcile these anta-gonisms in a coherent model which takes as given the interpenetrations and co-dependency of sexism and heterosexism?

LESBIANS IN WOMEN'S STUDIES – DIFFERENCE AND MARGINALISATION

Lesbian studies shares with women's studies more than the common gender 'female' (though there are those, such as Monique Wittig, who insist that even that is open to debate). Lesbian studies, like women's studies, is resolutely multi-disciplinary. The nature of lesbian oppression is characterised by a daunting ubiquity: 'lesbian' as a stigmatised 'other' has been constructed within a multiplicity of discourses and genres and the enterprise of deconstruction entails intervention within medicine, psychology, biology, socio-biology, sociology, art history, literary studies, history, linguistics, politics, social policy, education, Black Studies, cultural studies and feminism itself (the list is not exhaustive). Additionally, the recognition of lesbian existence and the articulation of a lesbian voice tends to disrupt the unquestioningly heterocentric practices of the academy, within whatever disciplinary context. Once 'lesbian' is recognised as a speaking/reading position rather than a mere object of study, then theory and practice predicated upon heterosexuality as the absolute norm and universal referent simply cease to be adequate.

This displacement is more radical than the paradigmatic shift catalysed by feminism. In the postmodern academy the totalitarian narrative of heterobinarism has yet to be deconstructed/decentred in the way that cultural androcentrism is being deconstructed by and within feminism. And lesbians, being marked as 'other' by reason of sexual practice as much as gender, are implicated in the disruptions of Queer as well as those of feminism. Since feminism depends upon heteropolarity as its foundational narrative, lesbian studies poses as radical a challenge to feminist academic praxis as it does to the malestream.

Heteropolar feminism is inadequate to the task of ending male supremacy. Unless lesbian-ness is always and everywhere recognised as a possibility, the apparatus of women's subordination remains invisible and unchallenged. For it is an apparatus which, as radical feminism recognises, deploys both gender and *the erotic* in the maintenance of its hegemony. This is a typical passage of feminist commentary:

> Disabled women put much more thought and effort into planning and pursuing social intercourse and are more dependent on their success than disabled men, who can rely on their wives in this respect. . . . Younger women, suffering from chronic sickness, disability or deformity, have to face the additional social disadvantage of being regarded as less valuable and desirable on the 'marriage market'.
>
> (Miles 1991: 111)

What Miles is describing, though failing to recognise that she is doing so, are the pressures which *heterosexuality* forces upon disabled women. In refusing to identify her 'women' and 'men' as *heterosexual*, she is colluding with the naturalisation of heterosexual gender relations which plays such an important role in women's subordination. A lesbian reading brings the precise politics of her (erased) critique into sharp focus. Thus, while *heterosexual* men may 'depend on their wives', gay men may not. We may therefore assume that somewhere in our society *now*, not in some feminist Utopia, there exist men who are quite different from the 'men' of this piece, men who demonstrate in their daily lives that it is possible for 'men' to do what *heterosexual* men are able to refuse to do because it is 'natural' for 'the wives' to manage their families' social world.

It is also quite absurd to suggest that 'women' share one position relative to the 'marriage market'. While a young disabled lesbian may just as easily find herself confronting rejection from potential sexual partners, she has no investment in 'the marriage market'.

Reading-as-lesbian in this strategic way adds an acuity and political maturity to non-lesbian feminist theory, which it otherwise lacks.[2] However, feminism has itself been a site for the construction of oppressive and stigmatising meanings around lesbianism and, far from being integrated into programmes of women's studies, lesbian studies has been at best marginalised/tokenised, at worst completely ignored (Franklin and Stacey 1986, Wilton 1993a).

Sadly, mainstream heterosexual feminism remains as hostile to lesbians and lesbian politics as in the 'gay/straight split' days of the 1960s. Although lesbians are as important to feminist research and scholarship as any other group of women, most feminist writers and academics seem oblivious to our very existence. An alarming majority of important feminist books ignore lesbian-ness entirely.[3] There is a particularly extraordinary trend for heterosexual feminists writing on sexuality to dispense with lesbians altogether by misnaming heterosexuality as sexuality,[4] and hostility to lesbians is freely expressed in some surprising quarters.[5]

Historically, then, feminism has served lesbians poorly and reluctantly, and feminist scholarship reinforces the unquestioned hegemony of heteropatriarchy by refusing to reflect on its own practice and, hence, colluding with the invisibility of lesbians (Jeffreys 1989). Patriarchal culture keeps all women, particularly lesbians, in ignorance of our history and our common interest and polices the sexuality and independence of all women by stigmatising lesbian sex. To collude with this is grossly anti-feminist as well as anti-lesbian. It is true that established women's studies courses do sometimes include lesbian material or provide a supportive framework within which lesbian studies can take place, but in my experience this only happens when out lesbian academics are able and willing to insist on it. Feminism in general, and women's studies in particular, have not been supportive and welcoming environments for lesbian students, lesbian teachers or lesbian studies.

FEMALE HOMOSEXUALS – ARE WE ALL QUEER TOGETHER?

Lesbian and gay/queer studies, although undoubtedly still far from mainstream, has been established for some time in the USA. The US Gay Academic Union has been in existence since March 1973, there is an Institute of Lesbian Studies at Pao Alto, California, and the Center for Lesbian and Gay Studies (CLAGS) in the City University of New York published a 196-page *Directory of Lesbian and Gay Studies* in 1994. In 1989, Columbia University Press initiated the first scholarly book series devoted to lesbian and gay studies, *Between Men, Between Women*. As an academic enterprise, lesbian and gay studies has achieved a firm base in the European mainland, with the establishment of such initiatives as the Interdisciplinary Gay and Lesbian Studies Department at the University of Utrecht, which publishes the Utrecht series on lesbian and gay studies and regularly organises conferences.

Even in Britain, lesbian and gay studies is slowly starting to grow. Lesbian and gay studies conferences take many forms – film studies, language studies, historical studies, sociology – and are well attended. One such, 'The Past and Future of Lesbian and Gay Studies', held at the University of Essex in 1991, gave rise to a *UK Directory of Lesbian and Gay Studies*. The prestigious British Sociological Association Annual Conference for 1994 was on the theme *Sexualities in Social Context*, and foregrounded queer issues. Publishers have launched new queer lists, from Virago's *Lesbian Landmarks* series to the up-front *Queer Sex* and *Women on Women* collections from Cassell. Does this blossoming enterprise offer lesbian studies a more welcoming and supportive 'home' than women's studies does?

Lesbian and gay studies and its love-child queer theory are newcomers to the academy, so any attempt to assess the potential benefits for lesbian studies must be based on informed guesswork. There can be no doubt that gay male scholars and writers have so far demonstrated a greater awareness of lesbian issues and a greater commitment to avoid marginalising lesbian work than heterosexual feminist scholars and writers have done (see, for example, Duberman *et al.* 1991, Dyer 1990). However, the privileges afforded men under heteropatriarchy are available to gay men *qua* men and, however much a few politically aware gay men may try to refuse the cultural imperative of masculinity, the inequalities between women and men are as much a shaping force of the lesbian and gay community[6] as of mainstream heterosexual society.

The contemporary queer/lesbian and gay subcultural infrastructure is dominated by economically privileged gay men. The greater part of the lesbian and gay press, including magazines such as *The Advocate* or *Gay Times*, is run by and for gay men, although a small and important lesbian press has been long established in the States and is making inroads into the British magazine market with publications such as *Diva*. The most important lesbian publisher in Britain, Onlywomen Press, is, in the words of its publicity, 'Radical Lesbian-Feminist', and avowedly hostile to self-styled 'sex-radical' lesbian-ness, so the choice for lesbian writers seeking publication outwith the commercial mainstream is between gay male publishing houses antagonistic towards feminism or feminist presses antagonistic towards many strands of Queer politics. It was Gay Men's Press, for example, who published Della Grace's book *Love Bites* (1991), which included sexualised lesbian images.

For lesbians of colour, the experience of homophobia from both whites and people of colour may not be separated from the daily realities of racism from both gays and straights. Many publish their work through specialist independent companies such as Kitchen Table Women of Colour Press.

ALLIES WITHIN ACADEME?

Within the academy, men and masculinist discourse maintain a familiar hegemony. Historically, the study of 'homosexuality' has been dominated by the study of *male* homosexuality as the paradigmatic 'norm of deviance' by which, if at all, the female was to be measured and defined. This is hardly surprising: lesbians are women, and women have been effectively 'written out' of the academy, whether as scholar or object of study, for centuries (Lesbian History Group 1989). Lesbian oppression is characterised by 'lesbian invisibility', denial of the reality, significance or existence of lesbians and lesbian relationships. Many lesbian books have titles which speak of the struggle to gain recognition of the baseline fact of lesbian existence: Martha Barron Barrett's (1990) *Invisible Lives*, Julia Penelope and Sarah Valentine's (1990) *Finding the*

Lesbians, the Hall Carpenter Archives Lesbian Oral History Group's (1989) collection *Inventing Ourselves*,[7] the National Lesbian and Gay Survey's (1992) *What a Lesbian Looks Like*.

Additionally, men continue to dominate the academic world. The number of influential women has doubtless increased, but such women are a minority in what is still very much a man's world. A gay man, whether open or closeted, is thus far more likely than a lesbian to be in a position to develop new curricula, get work published or obtain research funding, since his gender is more significant than his sexual preference. This is not, of course, to deny that being openly gay (or even being open about a concern for gay issues) is enough to shut doors and hold back a career, but it is important to recognise that the lesbian academic is under double jeopardy and that her sex is as much (if not more) of an obstacle than her sexuality.

For lesbian studies there is no pre-existing academic base. Women's studies is dogged by heterosexism, gay studies by sexism. A struggle for recognition, validation, credibility and resources is likely within either field. With the often contradictory demands of its dual nature (as stigmatised erotic practice and as political catalyst within feminist practice and theory), lesbian studies is a complex and uneasy presence within the pedagogic paradigm. Lesbian-ness, even more than feminism or male homosexuality, acts to subvert the assumptions and practices of the academy itself. Within all this complexity and contradiction, exactly what does lesbian studies consist of? Several interwoven strands may be identified crossing, in a typically irreverent way, disciplinary boundaries.

A TENTATIVE SYLLABUS FOR LESBIAN STUDIES

I would suggest that there are currently five major endeavours which may usefully be included under the heading of lesbian studies. All will be considered in greater detail later on in this book, but I outline them here to give some shape to the idea of lesbian studies.

1 Affirmation

Faced with a culture which derides and denies lesbianism, it has clearly been crucial, both in the context of what may be thought of as 'post-Stonewall'[8] lesbian and gay politics and in the context of feminism, to reclaim lesbian history.

Research into lesbian lives and into different attitudes towards lesbianism in different cultures and at different historical periods has taken place within both the larger feminist project of reclaiming women's history and gay scholarship recovering what has been erased from history. Much has been published as a result of this work, including biographies of well-known lesbians such as the painter Gluck or accounts of communities such as the American expatriate lesbians living in Paris in the first half of the twentieth century.

Researching a lesbian 'ancestry' is not comparable to researching Black ancestry or Jewish ancestry. Discovering what lesbians were doing in nineteenth-century England does not have the significance for a contemporary English lesbian that discovering the history of her African antecedents would have for an African-American woman. To speak of lesbians and gay men as 'a people', in the way that Jews or Romanies are a people, is clearly problematic, but evidence of previous generations of lesbians is nevertheless profoundly empowering in the face of a culture which denies lesbian reality.

It also gives rise to more important and unsettling theoretical questions. To what extent can 'lesbian' be used as an historical constant? Is it possible to use the word even for women living in the early part of our own century and know that the word meant then what it means now? Is the 'lesbian' of Djuna Barnes the same as the 'lesbian' of Pat Parker? Such questions, familiar in the context of contemporary historicity, which recognises the contingency of social roles and of moral, legal and religious concepts, begin to unsettle our certainty about something fondly presumed to be a basic and fundamental aspect of human nature – sexuality itself.

2 Theoretical critiques of sexuality

The strand of queer theory which seems to have leapt ahead of the mainstream to form a true intellectual avant-garde and which seems to have had most impact on scholarship in general is its deconstruction of gender and the unpacking of the entire field of sexuality. Michel Foucault has, of course, been central here, though he has been criticised for ignoring the role of gender in his analysis of the deployment of sexuality and the operation of power which inheres in it. The relationships among sexual identity, sexual desire and sexual behaviour have been problematised as a result of lesbian and gay social-historical research. Feminists first identified heterosexuality as a social construct deployed in order to maintain the subordination of women (Radicalesbians 1970, Rich 1981a), and Queer owes an (acknowledged) debt to feminism.

The work informed by a deconstructive critique of gender and the erotic ranges over a broad area. Important to lesbian studies have been debates around psychoanalysis, essentialism, social constructionism and historical/cultural relativism, and much has been published in these areas. A lesbian studies perspective is a particularly useful one from which to approach these debates, since 'lesbian' is the only available position outside the social and semiotic forcefield of phallocentric hetero-relations.

3 Feminism and lesbianism: theory and practice

Of course there is a rich lode of scholarship within lesbian feminism, and the interaction of lesbians with feminism has been a productive one. While it is important to recognise that there is more to lesbianism and lesbian studies than lesbian feminism, there can be no doubt that feminism catalysed the rupture of 'lesbian' from its ascribed identification with (heterosexual) masculinity, and was responsible for a dramatic flowering of lesbian culture and political theory. Radical feminism insists that lesbianism is political and that women who withhold their sexual and emotional energies from men and share them with women are making a powerful feminist statement. They point out that heterosexual women, being emotionally and sexually dependent on men, can never commit themselves 100 per cent to feminism, and that a lesbian – by definition as independent of men as it is possible to be – represents both a challenge to male power and a committed bedrock for the feminist struggle. This position is challenging both to heterosexual feminists and non-feminist lesbians, and there have been bitter struggles waged over political lesbianism. Lesbian feminism has been among the most active and productive sites of lesbian struggle and has resulted in a proliferation of stimulating and energetic debates. Feminism is an important part of lesbian studies.

4 Lesbian cultural studies

It has been important for feminists to recognise the instrumentality of representation in the construction of subjectivity and in the reflection and reproduction of male supremacy. Feminist scholars have also worked to restore and re-evaluate the work of women artists throughout history and to explain both why so few women appear to have achieved great stature in the arts and why their work has so often been belittled, denied and buried by male art historians (Greer 1979, Parker and Pollock

1981, Petersen and Wilson 1976). In addition to the art historical and cultural deconstructionist work being done by feminist scholars, there has also been a blossoming of feminist and feminist-inspired cultural production. Women's participation in elite and popular culture has become a site of struggle, as women's work has proliferated in galleries, concert halls, libraries, cinemas and theatres. The divide between the 'fine' and 'minor' arts has been problematised and identified as a strategy of male supremacy, and traditional female arts such as embroidery, weaving and china-painting have been reclaimed and re-evaluated.[9] A strong feminist tradition has developed in literary studies in particular, establishing new sets of critical and reading practices.

Similar processes have been taking place among lesbians. Lesbian cultural studies has debated such issues as: Is there a lesbian gaze; a lesbian voice in literature, in music; a specific lesbian sensibility? What are the processes and strategies of lesbian spectatorship in the context of hegemonic heterosexuality and the objectification of women in/by main-stream cultural production? What are the politics of representation of lesbian issues; of lesbian sexuality and sexual practices? How does lesbian reading engage with and make meaning of texts? Simultane-ously, the lesbian community has been producing affirmative lesbian culture. Lesbian silversmiths, designers, song-writers, playwrights, poets, novelists, potters, artists, cartoonists, photographers and musicians have been using their skills to record and celebrate lesbian existence. Engag-ing both in an on-going critique of culture from a lesbian perspective and in a critique of specifically lesbian culture is an important part of lesbian studies.

5 The social sciences – lesbian subject, lesbian object

Sociology and social policy are both important areas of study for the scholar with an interest in lesbian issues. Social policy debates concerning employment rights, parenting, education, health and equal opportunities issues in general are of very real importance in the lives of lesbian women, and the knowledge and skills needed to challenge the making and implementation of social policy are essential survival skills, as they are for all oppressed groups. Political awareness, in a local, national and international context, is essential both to an understanding of the many meanings of lesbian at this point in time and to the struggle for lesbian rights.

Traditional heterosexual sociology has adopted an anthropological approach to lesbians (and gay men) as representative of a culture, almost a species, which is entirely 'other' to the curious or disgusted voyeurism of the dominant heterosexual group. Increasingly, accounts of lesbian and gay life and culture are being published by lesbians and gay men themselves, though very little sociological research by lesbians for lesbians is currently available, and almost none which goes beyond the collection of and reflection on life stories or coming-out stories. This is an area which invites greater attention, since the social sciences, with their insights into social processes such as stigma and deviance, the deployment of power and the reproduction of hegemonic norms, are clearly of key importance for lesbian studies.

Of importance, too, is a lesbian studies of social policy. Making clear the position of lesbians *vis-à-vis* the state and the apparatus of public power is of obvious significance. Here, gender and erotic identity interweave in the relationship of lesbians to the Welfare State, to the economy, to education, health care, the labour market and – perhaps most powerfully – the family.

SOME PROBLEMS AND QUESTIONS

Many of the unsettling questions which beset lesbian studies have long been problematic for women's studies, too, though others are specific to lesbian studies. It is clearly not possible to cover them all in detail here, and many will be discussed at greater length in other chapters, but some key themes are introduced here.

Essentialism

Essentialism has been one of the most vexing problems for women's studies and is proving still more so for lesbian studies. The problem for women's studies (and, more widely, for feminist political strategy) has been that, since the goal of feminism is to deconstruct and finally dispense with any form of social stratification predicated upon gender, it is counter-productive and illogical to subscribe to academic practices which privilege precisely a demarcation along lines of gender.

For lesbian studies the problem of essentialism is still more acute, as lesbian identity itself is now widely accepted as being culturally and historically contingent and, moreover, as being shaped largely in reaction to oppression. There are also the fundamental questions of sexual difference, sexual practice, sexual desire and sexual identity, all of which have profound strategic and intellectual significance.[10] The very act of declaring that there is such a thing as lesbian studies contributes powerfully to the reification of 'the lesbian' as a distinct and identifiable creature, something which runs counter to current radical theories of sexuality. Questions of definition are thorny. Whether we subscribe to Rich's continuum model of lesbian-ness, to a 'lesbian' as a discrete sub-group of 'women' (Rich 1981a) or to a Queer lesbian outwith the heterosexual binary of gender altogether, dictates where we may locate the boundary between lesbian studies and women's studies. Since 'lesbian' stands in such volubly contested relation to 'woman', lesbian studies may be able to maintain intellectual consistency only by evolving a permeable and shifting praxis.

Aetiology

There exists a disease model of lesbianism which is quite distinct from the more general pathologising of women that has been identified by feminist writers (Doyal 1995, Doyal and Elston 1986, Laws *et al.* 1985, Showalter 1985), and hence there is an over-riding emphasis within traditional academic practice on explaining the origin or cause of lesbianism, in order that it may be prevented or cured. The disease model postulates an aetiology (lesbianism is supposedly caused by any number of factors, including psychological trauma, pre-natal exposure to the 'wrong' mix of hormones, neural pathology or chromosomal abnormality), a symptomatology (there is great anxiety expressed generally about how one may recognise a lesbian, and symptoms of lesbianism proposed by the medical industry have included irregular menstruation, excess body/facial hair, enlarged clitoris and suicidal tendencies!) and therapy (historically including pre-frontal lobotomy, aversion therapy, etc.), and there is much anxiety about the possibility of infection or contagion.

The consequences of the disease model of lesbianism are wide ranging, the most important being the drive to study lesbianism as an abnormality rather than as a social role or a political role. In the social sciences, for example, lesbianism itself rather than homophobia has been seen as the object of enquiry. The disease paradigm demands to be confronted unequivocally, since it is clearly obstructive to a lesbian studies, which takes the 'health' of lesbian-ness as given.

Ghettoisation

Deciding on the best position for lesbian studies is not easy. The philosophy and political strategy of separatism claims that working in safe lesbian space, removed from contact with the daily pain and drain of heterosexist oppression, is a necessity. Others question this strategy, seeing it as self-defeating isolationism. There can be no doubt that the most brilliant scholarly or political work, if carried out in isolation, cannot hope to engage adequately with or develop an informed and influential critique of mainstream thinking. Equally, there can be no doubt that the demands made on lesbians, as on members of any oppressed minority group within the academy, both in terms of sheer survival and in the assumption that they should contribute to the enlightenment and education of the majority about their own oppression, put an unfair burden on lesbian students and teachers. This is a powerful argument in favour of at least a degree of separate provision for lesbian learning, whether within the mainstream academy or within the lesbian community. As this book makes clear, I think the academy needs lesbian studies if anything rather *more* urgently than lesbian studies needs the academy.

Objectification

Whether within women's studies or within more traditional academic disciplines, lesbians are likely to find themselves the object of scholarly curiosity. An anxiety-provoking deviation from the sexual norm, lesbianism has been the object of proliferating descriptive and explanatory endeavour, more or less offensive, across the discursive practices of almost every academic field of study. Like moths on a pin, lesbians have been subjected to the scrutiny of endocrinologists, human biologists, neurologists, sexologists, sociobiologists, sociologists, behavioural scientists, psychologists, psychiatrists, anthropologists, historians, feminists, literary critics and cineastes (the list is not exhaustive). Every aspect of a lesbian's life, from her intelligence to the size and shape of her genitals, from her childhood to her sexual practices, from her eating habits to her politics, has been described, assessed, theorised and manipulated to suit the purposes of heterosexual supremacy.

The result of all this is that for lesbian scholars the feminist doctrine that the personal is political becomes a lived experience. For lesbians, there is never any respite from *being studied*, whether as part of a formal syllabus or simply as the object of idle curiosity. This is a problem for lesbian studies where, by definition, the object of study is lesbian-ness and lesbian issues. Similar difficulties face women's studies, where work around domestic violence, child abuse, mental health and other issues of central concern to feminism frequently intersect painfully with the lived experience of students, teachers and researchers. Where the situation of lesbians differs from that of heterosexual women in this situation is that issues such as rape and domestic violence do not involve the construction of a sub-group of women seen as radically different from women as a whole. Within the women's studies classroom the lesbian is marked as 'other' as powerfully as she is in malestream discourse. This otherness has much in common with race/colour or disability (all vectors of difference which may, of course, intersect in one individual). What separates 'lesbian' from 'Black' or 'disabled', however, is a set of instabilities around behaviour/essence, visibility/passing, legality/illegality, fixedness/conversion, all compounded by the anxiety-provoking fact that 'lesbian' is in some sense 'about' sex and the erotic.

Marginalisation

Lesbian studies must not be allowed to collapse into a ghetto. All academic subject areas, all textual and pedagogic practices, need to set their own house in order as far as lesbian issues are concerned. Oppressive and offensive constructions of lesbianism are present across disciplinary boundaries, and must be eradicated. There is precious little to be gained from ground-breaking work in lesbian studies if psychology is still tilling the sterile soil of penis envy or if sociobiology continues to maintain that women's desire for women is programmed into their selfish genes. Given the anxious insularity with which the academy polices disciplinary boundaries, it is probable that the existence of lesbian studies as a visible entity would give far too many academics the excuse they are looking for to avoid dealing with lesbian criticisms of their particular subject area.

However, there are practical advantages in such a strategy. Current developments in higher and further education in Britain and elsewhere, with education being seen more and more in classical liberal terms as a mere commodity subject to the unrestrained demands of the open market, mean that the law of supply and demand dictates a proliferation of discrete areas of study, short courses, non-traditional award routes, etc. Within such a climate there are undoubted advantages to be gained from establishing an identifiable academic base, from which strategic interventions in other areas may be made, and to which other practitioners look for guidance, academic excellence and archival support.

Much important work in lesbian studies takes place in adult education, continuing education, community education, etc. For many lesbians, such courses represent their only opportunity for further education in this area and are perceived as less likely to discriminate against lesbians, working-class women or women of colour. They are, and will remain, a vital resource for lesbians. It is in the relationship between work of this nature and the more formal academic work in universities that marginalisation is potentially most destructive. Only by an active and vigorous exchange across the boundaries of 'further' and 'higher' education can lesbian studies succeed in establishing a firm academic base while remaining accessible to and stimulated by the very community from which it grew.

CONCLUSION – FOR NOW

Lesbian studies is a complex, amorphous and *shifting* entity. In the process of developing a distinct academic infrastructure, it must also remain accessible to and supportive of the grass roots lesbian community. It must provide a safe and stimulating learning environment for lesbian students, teachers and researchers, while at the same time challenging heterosexist bias and anti-lesbianism in the academy more generally. It must offer support to lesbians, foreground lesbian issues and contribute a lesbian perspective, while simultaneously deconstructing notions of lesbian identity. It should encompass affirmation of lesbian existence and of lesbian cultural production, whilst at the same time engaging in radical critiques of sexuality and sociological explorations of heterosexism, stigma and the disciplinary power that accrues to both. It has a crucial contribution to make to theory and activism in the context of feminism and queer, and must resist incorporation and marginalisation within either. It is vigorously multi-disciplinary, and must facilitate a paradigmatic shift of focus within and between a multitude of discourses. It is the purpose of this book to offer a starting point for this extraordinarily broad enterprise.

NOTES

1 Feminists have been saying this for a very long time. Charlotte Perkins Gilman, wrote her book *The Man-Made Word or Our Androcentric Culture*, published by T. Fisher Unwin in 1911; Mary Beard in 1931 wrote an article in *Independent Woman*, vol. 10 no. 8 entitled 'Women at the Crossroads', and Virginia Woolf's famous work *Three Guineas* was first published in 1938.
2 My women's studies students never fail to be delighted and astonished by the fresh light shed on familiar feminist themes by this strategy. Try it for a week . . .

3   Important feminist texts which ignore the issue of lesbianism include; Juliet
    Mitchell and Ann Oakley (1976) *The Rights and Wrongs of Women*, Barbara
    Ehrenreich and Dierdre English (1979) *For Her Own Good* and Pamela
    Abbott and Claire Wallace (1990) *An Introduction to Sociology: Feminist
    Perspectives*. Classic texts like Germaine Greer's *The Female Eunuch*, first
    published in 1971, or Shulamith Firestone's *The Dialectic of Sex* (1970)
    either ignore lesbians entirely or, in the case of Firestone, insist that 'Homo-
    sexuals in our time are only the extreme casualties of the system of obstructed
    sexuality that develops in the family' (Firestone 1970: 61). It is, even now,
    almost unheard of for a non-lesbian feminist writer to discuss lesbianism
    with any degree of acceptance or awareness. Cynthia Cockburn and Patricia
    Hill Collins spring to mind as among the few honourable exceptions.
4   Thus Annette Kuhn (1988) *Cinema, Censorship and Sexuality 1909–1925*
    and Carol Smart's (1992) *Regulating Womanhood: Marriage, Motherhood
    and Sexuality*, although purporting to deal with sexuality in fact confine
    themselves to *hetero*sexuality, while Mary O'Brien's (1981) *The Politics of
    Reproduction* contrives to maintain absolute silence on the subject of les-
    bianism. It is difficult to understand how it could be possible to theorise
    censorship, the regulation of female sexuality or the patriarchal control of
    reproduction without a critique of compulsory heterosexuality. Such
    narrowness surely makes for inadequate scholarship.
5   For example, Marsha Hunt's (1990) novel *Joy* and Maya Angelou's (1971)
    Gather Together in My Name both contain extremely offensive lesbian
    stereotypes, while Julia Neuberger speaks of lesbian feminism as 'very
    damaging to the feminist cause' (1991: 23). Maud Sulter, writing about a
    celebration of Black women's art in her book *Passion: Discourses on
    Blackwomen's Creativity*, casually mentions 'Lioness Chant caused con-
    sternation with an anti-lesbian poem' (Sulter 1990: 16). The relative
    acceptance accorded anti-lesbian sentiment is revealed when one considers
    what the response would be to anti-working class, anti-Black, anti-disabled
    or anti-woman poetry.
6   I use the terms 'lesbian and gay community' or 'gay community' in the full
    knowledge that the notion of a community among lesbians and gay men is
    a problematic one. However, I believe it is important to recognise that there
    do exist loose networks of lesbian and gay peoples both within individual
    towns/cities/countries and organising around specific issues (such as
    HIV/AIDS or cultural activism), as well as what might be described as an
    international lesbian and gay network. The support and strength created by
    this community or set of communities are essential both for the self-esteem
    and happiness of individual lesbians and gay men and for the struggle for
    lesbian and gay rights. I owe much to my membership of this 'community'
    and, for all its inaccuracy and clumsiness as a term, for all that it disguises
    crucial sets of difference, it still has important meanings.
7   Of course, as the astute reader will point out, *Hidden from History*, an
    account of lesbian *and gay* history, is just such a title. There are undeniably
    similarities between the ways in which gay men's and lesbians' histories
    have been erased, hidden and denied. There are, however, issues around
    invisibility and denial which are specific to lesbians because they are
    women. These will be discussed further in the next chapter.

8 'Stonewall' refers to the incident identified by many lesbian and gay scholars and commentators as the beginning of the modern gay rights movement. On 27 June 1969 police raided the Greenwich Village gay bar, the Stonewall Inn. Such raids were commonplace, but on this occasion lesbians and gay men (fronted up, many accounts suggest, by drag queens and effeminate gay men) rebelled in outrage and rioted for four nights, inspiring in lesbians and gay men around the world a new spirit of militancy and a refusal to be intimidated.

9 The most famous example of traditional 'feminine' craftwork being re-cuperated for/as art is Judy Chicago's installation 'The Dinner Party'. Chicago produced two books detailing the collective process of creating this gargantuan work in which ecclesiastical and traditional folk embroid-ery techniques were used alongside china-painting and innovative clay sculptural methods to produce an installation honouring and celebrating the life and work of thirty-nine significant women from history.

10 For an outline of the many debates relating to sexual identity see Dennis Altman *et al.* (1989) *Which Homosexuality? Essays from the International Scientific Conference on Lesbian and Gay Studies*, published by the Gay Men's Press.

Chapter 2

The nature of the beast
What is a lesbian?

Because it forced itself upon me I told the absence-of-signifier theory
of women to get knotted. It was.

(Lahire 1987: 276)

A less essentialising view of experience would recognise its
construction in ideological practices, allowing for the expression,
perhaps, of essentialist moments as an expedient political trajectory.

(Munt 1992: xvi)

NATURE, ESSENCE, THING?

Arriving at a working definition of 'lesbian' is fraught with difficulty
and contradiction, there is no consensus about what defines or even what
characterises a lesbian. The word is variously understood and positioned
within a multiplicity of paradigms: the moral, the mystical/religious, the
juridical, the scientific, the medical, the political and the social.
'Lesbianism' can mean immoral behaviour, a sin, a crime, a sexual
perversion, a pathological state, a site of or metaphor for resistance, a
form of deviance or a social role/lifestyle. Among lesbians ourselves
there is profound dissensus about lesbian identity, with essentialist and
constructionist theories of varying kinds and degrees giving rise to
contradictory and often competing performances of 'lesbian', as well as
political and theoretical positions. Additionally, 'lesbian', in common
with all other social identities, is open to a particular kind of theoretical
dispersal within and by means of the deconstructionist idiom of
postmodernism.

'Lesbian' is not an extra-social entity transcendent of the historical
and/or the cultual. To recognise that evidence of sexual activity between
women exists across cultures and through history is not to say that there

were/are *lesbians* in dynastic Egypt, pre-Columbian America, Neanderthal Europe or contemporary China, who require only to be uncovered by sympathetic research. Nor does existing evidence support the general view of lesbianism as a 'condition' pertaining to specific individuals, comparable to being tall or to having Down's syndrome. Rather, lesbian-ness is a product of the shifting relationships among individual subjectivity, the body and the social (including kinship networks, sub-cultural groups, etc.), and of meanings constituted by/within those relationships. Such relationships are characterised by activity and rapid change, with the result that 'lesbian' is a word in constant flux, subject to continual negotiation and renegotiation. Diane Richardson describes how one direction of this intrinsically dialectical process works:

> The process whereby a woman identifies as a lesbian or not, and (if she does) the meaning and significance such an identification will have for her, will be influenced by the wider social meanings ascribed to lesbianism that she encounters, as well as the specific response of significant others to this information.
>
> (Richardson 1981: 112)

This semiotic process is not unidirectional – modifications and reassessments occur within the sign 'lesbian' in various discourses in reponse to the performative lesbianisms of individual women and sub-cultural groups. Indeed, catalysing such modifications has traditionally been the political aim of homophile activism (Faderman 1991).

Richardson goes on to identify four commonalities which she perceives in prevailing (heterosexual) accounts of lesbians: that they are pseudo-males; that lesbianism is a 'sorry state to be in'; that it is a permanent condition; and that lesbianism may be defined primarily in relation to sex (she includes within this both accounts which perceive lesbians as too sexual, and hence 'morally dangerous', and contradictory ones which insist that lesbians are not sexual enough). To these I would add other themes which crop up with varying degrees of regularity in oppositional accounts of lesbian-ness: that 'lesbian' functions to disrupt the articulacy of gender as an ontological category or socio-sexual framework; that it is intrinsically feminist–political; that lesbian-ness is no more than a social construct, having no extra-social reality; and that to *be* lesbian is 'more than a sexual identity'. Clearly, these assertions interact with one another in a kind of alchemical reaction, each functioning to support/disrupt the others, constantly pre-empting the semantic stability of 'lesbian'.

The only strategy which enables us to make sense of the semantic conundrum in which 'lesbian' is embedded is to replace the traditional focus on lesbianism with 'an ethnography of societal reactions to same-sex experience' (Plummer 1981b). This chapter adopts this strategy, interrogating various discursive accounts of 'lesbian' in order to expose the dialectical mechanisms at work in what is clearly a politics of naming.

THE MEDICAL MODEL

Perhaps the most familiar set of assertions about lesbians are those of the 'founding fathers' of the modern lesbian identity, the sexologists and psychologists whose taxonomic enthusiasm gave birth to the homosexual (and the heterosexual) of both sexes (Faderman 1991, Foucault 1976, Weeks 1977/1990). For it is within what we may broadly term the medical model that sexual desires and acts were first pressed into service as the definitional characteristics of distinct types of people (see Chapter 4 for more detailed discussion of this). From the mid-nineteenth century up until the present day, the privileged definition of 'lesbian' is located in models of pathology (whether physiological or psychological). In popular terms, 'these people are sick'. As the following comments show, adherents to the medical model go to sometimes farcical lengths to pathologise 'lesbian'.

> Homosexuality is a symptom of neurosis and of a grievous personality disorder. It is an outgrowth of deeply rooted emotional deprivations and disturbances that had their origins in infancy. It is manifested, all too often, by compulsive and destructive behaviour that is the very antithesis of fulfillment and happiness. Buried under the 'gay' exterior of the homosexual is the hurt and rage that cripples his or her capacity for true maturation, for healthy growth and love.
>
> (Kronemeyer 1980, in Kitzinger 1987: 40)

This account betrays its counter-liberationist agenda by its refutation of the word 'gay' as appropriate to describe 'homosexuals'. Its central assertion, that same-sex desire is only a *symptom* marking the underlying pathology of destructive, unhappy, immature and disturbed individuals, was at the time of writing already rendered obsolete by numerous research findings (see Ruse 1988). However, Kronemeyer clearly feels impelled to insist that homosexuality is very bad news indeed. The very stridency of his argument – 'hurt', 'rage', 'cripples', 'neurosis', 'grievous', 'disorder', 'deprivations', 'disturbances', 'destructive', 'compulsive' are all powerfully negative words and all appear within four short sentences – strongly suggests not cool scientific commentary but the over-determined emotionality of anxious repudiation.

The anxiety to repudiate and invalidate lesbian desire does not stop at making unverifiable claims about what is 'really' going on inside people's heads. It leads supposedly level-headed scientists to mutate observable somatic bodies in a wildly improbable manner. Thus:

> Frank Caprio, M.D., states not only that some lesbians have 'an unusually elongated' clitoris but provides the datum of 'about six centimetres,' while the ever knowledgeable David Reuben, M.D., informs his public that a clitoris 'as much as two or more inches in length when erect' is possible and that 'lesbians with this anatomical quirk are very much in demand'.
>
> (Barale 1991)

As Susan Hemmings points out, such flights of fancy are far from benign:

> Sometimes this seemingly wilful ignorance leads to situations bordering on malpractice. A friend of mine had suffered for a long time with lumps in her breast and other worrying symptoms. One specialist finally stumbled on the fact of her lesbianism. He subsequently wrote to her GP saying that her problem was hormonal: as a lesbian she had 'an enlarged clitoris' and 'body hair'. In actual fact, just to put the record straight, she has neither.
>
> (Hemmings 1986)

This last anecdote should alert us to the fact that, however risible the contortions of homophobic 'science' may appear, there are real consequences for flesh-and-blood women who inhabit the lesbian body. Accounts oppositional to the above but which still predicate their authoritative voice on an acceptance of the normal/abnormal polarity so central to the medical model, insist on the absolute normality of the lesbian subject, of her 'sameness' as distinct from her 'otherness', in an attempt to win for the 'body normal' acceptance by the body politic: 'It is no longer clear . . . if a distinction now exists between homosexuals and heterosexuals' (Chesebro 1981). This normalisation project is particularly apparent in psychology:

> In reviewing my experiences with lesbian clients, I see them struggling with the same issues as other people. . . . There is no particular psychotherapy for lesbians, but, rather, psychotherapy for women who happen to be lesbians.
>
> (Anthony 1982)

Accounts such as these fail to challenge or disrupt the model of normality/ deviance which has historically been so powerful in the oppression of many marginalised groups. As several writers have commented, the trend of replacing homosexuality-as-pathology with homophobia-as-pathology achieves no more than a change of focus. As long as the notion of pathology remains available for political deployment, there can be no guarantee that the object of 'pathologification' will not one day again be lesbian or gay (Kitzinger 1987).

TOO SEXY, OR NOT SEXY ENOUGH?

Both within and outwith the medical model, several competing positions define 'lesbian' solely or mainly in terms of sexual activity and desire. The classic construction of the lesbian as female homosexual positions us on the spectrum of sexual perversions categorised by sexologists such as Westphahl, Ellis, Carpenter, etc. The challenge to this position mounted by homophile and feminist writers in the mid-twentieth century declared that sex is *not* the defining characteristic of lesbianism, while some radical lesbian-feminists see specific sexual *acts* as intrinsically *heterosexual*, independent of the gender of the actors, and therefore politically contaminating of a lesbian body, defined as the site of resistance *par excellence* to male power (see below pp. 99–101). This, in turn, has sparked resistance among other lesbians, who claim certain sexual practices as being transgressive and politically radical *per se*, and whose primary identification is with queers rather than feminists. The following extracts demonstrate the place of the erotic in competing definitions of 'lesbian'.

> LESBIAN: A woman who has sexual relationships with other women, and who may or may not participate in her gay culture.
>
> (Grahn 1984)

> There is a passion, or a perversion of appetite, which, like all human passions, has played a considerable part in the world's history for good or evil. . . . Inverted sexuality, the sexual instinct diverted from its normal channel . . .
>
> (Symonds 1840/1984)

> No female homosexual subjects were recruited who were not capable of attaining orgasm through masturbation, partner manipulation[1] and cunnilingus.
>
> (Masters and Johnson 1979)

[Lesbianism includes] a range – throughout each woman's life history of woman-identified experience; not simply the fact that a woman has had or consciously desired genital sexual experience with another woman.

(Rich 1981a)

A lesbian is a woman whose primary erotic, psychological, emotional and social interest is in members of her own sex, even though that interest may not be overtly expressed.

(Martin and Lyon 1972)

There are lesbians who have never had a sexual relationship with another woman, and there are women who have had sexual experiences with women but do not identify as lesbians.

(Rupp 1989)

A lesbian is a woman-identified woman who does not fuck men.

(Leeds Revolutionary Feminists 1981)

Women who like penetration may feel ambivalent about it and wonder if it isn't 'sort of heterosexual'. Any technique that two women use to arouse and please each other is a *lesbian* technique.

(Califia 1988)

It is clear that the sexological notion of *sexual identity* catalysed a vigorous and polyvocal set of contestations concerning the relationship between sex and a lesbian identity which is still very far from resolved. Do we define a lesbian as a woman who has sex exclusively with women, who prefers sex with women while still having sex with men, who desires and likes but does not have sex with women or who merely refuses to have sex with anybody, including men? Are there specific lesbian and non-lesbian sexual *acts*?

Equally problematic is the location of 'lesbian' relative to gender, to the 'necessary fictions' of masculine and feminine, and the insights this offers into the elision of eroticism and gender more widely.

MORE OF A MAN THAN YOU'LL EVER BE, MORE OF A WOMAN THAN YOU CAN HANDLE?

(Traditional response of butch lesbians to male baiting)

The medical model of lesbianism often blurs into the notion that lesbians are pseudo-males, a belief that takes many forms. Added to the old notion that a woman who desired women was *really* a man trapped in a woman's body is the Freudian idea that lesbians suffer from penis envy. Both reinsert the affronted/rejected penis into a sexual arena that dispenses with it, by claiming it as the longed-for potent *absence* in lesbian desire. As Simone de Beauvoir suspects, the totalitarianism of androcentrism leaves all women trapped in the fictions of male agency, sexual or otherwise: 'Whenever she behaves as a human being, she is declared to be identifying herself with the male' (de Beauvoir 1953).

It is this heteropolarising of the social and the erotic that makes Queer necessary. Queer activism shares with queer theory the will to destabilise gender as an ontological category and has self-consciously adopted to that end a parodic playfulness not only with male and female signifiers but also with specific erotic behaviours expressive of and definitional of *sexual* identity. It is not merely the male/female binary which is being perverted, but the homo/heterosexual, too. Thus the idea that lesbians are 'pseudo-men' has been co-opted in a reverse discourse which deconstructs the contextual/conceptual links between biological, social and erotic sex.

What Queer neglects to recognise is the significance of heteropolarity in maintaining male power. The traditional penis-deprivation model, expressed in the following passages from male writers, reveals with somewhat touching clarity the not-so-hidden agenda of male anxiety and the desperate need to colonise lesbianism for phallocentrism.

> Lesbians who protest that, for them, this kind of relationship is better than any possible intimacy with a man do not know what they are really missing.[2] There is no doubt that for women who, for whatever reason, have been unable to get married, a homosexual partnership may be a happier way of life than a frustrated loneliness, but this is not to say that it can ever fully satisfy.
>
> (Storr 1964)

> The case of female homosexuality is remarkably different. . . . There is not the same emphasis [as in male homosexuals] on the sexual organs and on the moment of sexual excitement; instead there is an extremely poignant, often helpless, sense of being at another's mercy. The lesbian knows that she desires someone who will not typically make those advances that are characteristic of a man, even if she wants to; nor can she make these advances herself without compromising the gender-identity which (she wishes to believe) is integral to her own attractiveness. She can only wait, and wish, and pray to the gods with . . . troubled fervour.
>
> (Scruton 1986)

In the face of the potentially threatening rejection of phallic power by lesbians, Scruton and Storr comfort themselves that this apparent rejection is not 'real'. By redefining lesbianism around the absence of the penis and constructing an imaginary lesbian subject humiliated, made miserable and sexually frustrated by this absence, they are able to reassure themselves that they have what all women, *even lesbians*, really need – a penis. In Victorian times, as this description of 'the lesbian' suggests, the cigarette or the microscope were as much signifiers of phallic masculinity as the fleshly penis:

> For female employments there is manifested not merely a lack of taste, but often unskillfulness in them. The toilette is neglected and pleasure found in coarse boyish life. Instead of an inclination for the arts, there is manifested an inclination and taste for the sciences. Occasionally there may be attempts to drink and smoke.
>
> (Kraft-Ebbing 1882, in Kitzinger 1987)

But it is not only within straightforward patriarchal discourse that the phallus functions as the logos of sexual desire. Some feminists, especially those who have attempted to reclaim psychoanalysis for feminism, have replicated as unproblematic the elision between the erotic and gender, constructing certain behaviours (sexual agency in particular) as intrinsically masculine and others (sexual passivity and responsiveness, narcissism) as intrinsically feminine. 'Lesbian', within this paradigm, is bound up with virility and with the primacy of male erotic agency.

> The convolutions involved here are analogous to those described by Julia Kristeva as 'the double or triple twists of what we commonly call female homosexuality. . . . I am looking, as a man would, for a woman; or else I submit myself, as if I were a man who thought he were a woman, to a woman who thinks she is a man.'
>
> (Doane 1987, in White 1991)

Even the anarchic exponents of gender-fuck end up playing in a rather docile fashion with categories which pre-exist their critique, as Cherry Smyth suggests when she asks, 'Do lesbians have to appropriate phallocentric images of sexuality in order to represent an active sexual arousal and autonomy because there is no such obvious symbol in lesbian sex?' (Smyth 1992). But, putting the semiotic revisionism of Queer aside, can 'lesbian' contain *any* coherent meaning within Queer?

> After years of saying those dildoes weren't really cocks, these lesbians are now letting everyone know that they like to suck cock, but

as lesbians – in the daddy/boy scene, a cock can be a tongue, fingers, a dildo, an idea, or an actual dick. It's not a retreat to something as obvious and straightforward as bisexuality. . . . Sure, the meaning of the word 'lesbian' is getting stretched a bit out of shape here.

(*Quim* 2 [1991])

Lesbians even have 'gay male' sex.

(Grace, in Smyth 1992)

Queer is a firework display of disobedience and eroticised transgression which has not yet developed an analysis of power capable of incorporating the key issues of racism, sexism, anti-semitism and body fascism so endemic to the lesbian and gay milieu, never mind a coherent deconstruction of gender. Because of this political inadequacy, its popular face has not moved much beyond a series of outrageous fashion statements (Burston 1992, Smyth 1992). It expresses a fundamental resistance to the taken-for-grantedness of gender, something which brings it into line with feminism. This is somewhat ironic, given that Queer has tended to assign bad-mummy status to feminism. But feminism has been the principle terrain within which the ontological stability of gender has been challenged:

Lesbian is the only concept I know which is beyond the categories of sex (woman and man), because the designated subject (lesbian) is *not* a woman . . . what makes a woman is a specific social relation to a man, a relation that we have previously called servitude, a relation which implies personal and physical obligation as well as economic obligation . . . a relation which lesbians escape by refusing to become or to stay heterosexual.

(Wittig 1981)

Lesbianism . . . is a category of behaviour possible only in a sexist society characterized by rigid sex roles and dominated by male supremacy. . . . In a society in which men do not oppress women, and sexual expression is allowed to follow feelings, the categories of homosexuality and heterosexuality would disappear. 'Lesbian' is one of the sexual categories by which men have divided up humanity.

(Radicalesbians 1970)

If the theoretical and political deconstruction of gender renders problematic the notion that anyone can *be* a woman (or a man), the exposure of the political nature of sexual identities similarly problematises the notion that anyone can *be* straight, gay or lesbian, while the radical lesbian feminism of Wittig merely removes lesbians from the category 'women' altogether. While the notion of gender/erotic performativity developed by queer academics such as Judith Butler (1990, 1993) sits easily with feminist gender-cynicism, it removes the political significance of 'lesbian' as a site of resistance to male power.

THE LESBIAN AS FEMINIST GUERILLA

It is within the multiplicity of feminisms that we find the most directly political definitions of 'lesbian', some of which, with Wittig, position lesbian outside gender while others insist that it is, on the contrary, the most privileged sign of womanliness. Where feminism differs from gay liberationist or Queer accounts of lesbianism is in its recognition of gender as the structure by means of which power is differentially assigned to men and to women.

> While both lesbians and gay men are not 'heterosexual', heterosexuality itself is a power relationship of men over women; what gay men and lesbians are rejecting are essentially polar experiences.
>
> (Faraday 1981)

> A lesbian is the rage of all women condensed to the point of explosion.
>
> (Radicalesbians 1970)

> Lesbianism is the practice and feminism is the theory.[3]
>
> (feminist slogan in Nestle 1987)

> The startling fact is that Lesbians already meet the criteria that Women's Liberation has set up to describe the liberated woman. . . . Lesbians have economic independence, sexual self-determination, that is, control over their own bodies and lifestyles. . . . Lesbians live what Feminists theorize about; they embody Feminism.
>
> (Abbott and Love 1972)

Ironically, feminists tend to position 'lesbian' in relation to men; as a woman who is defined precisely by means of her independence from men, her refusal to have sex with men. This approach at its most polemical is barely indistinguishable from the phallocentrism of Scruton and Storr, predicated as it is upon the definitional supremacy of the (absent) penis. The emphasis on woman-identification, often seen as a more liberal feminist position, appears in fact more radical, in that it refuses the penis such a powerful definitional status. It is probably only the 'lesbian' of Monique Wittig and the Radicalesbians, positioned *outside* the discursive structurations of gender and deployed by Wittig in order to map out a radically oppositional system of signifiers, which may be said to disrupt phallocentrism. This 'lesbian' is also the one most in tune with the deconstructionism of postmodern idiom.

A DYKE TO HOLD BACK THE SHIFTING SANDS OF POSTMODERNISM?

The postmodern socio-historical position on homosexuality is exemplified by writers such as Michel Foucault, Mary McIntosh, Carol Vance and Jeffrey Weeks. According to this model, sexual identities are historically and culturally contingent and, therefore, opaque to retrospective scrutiny. This position clearly owes much to the exposure by feminism of what were then generally called 'sex roles' as being socially constructed rather than natural and, in turn, has influenced the development of postmodern feminism (Tong 1989). Foucault notes the historical convergence of gender and the erotic:

> Homosexuality appeared as one of the forms of sexuality when it was transposed from the practice of sodomy onto a kind of anterior androgony, a hermaphrodism of the soul.
>
> (Foucault 1979)

Homosexuality (including, by definition, lesbianism, though Foucault has been justly criticised for his neglect of gender) is understood by Foucault as a construct delineated by, expressive of and maintaining the hegemony of the sets of beliefs and doctrines about sexual behaviour dominant at any one time and in any one place. The radical idea that homosexuality itself is an historically recent concept, and that in the past the behaviours we call homosexual have not necessarily been regarded as indicative of a discrete type of person, has been influential in determining current discursive constructs of 'homosexual' and 'lesbian'.

> One might as well try to trace the aetiology of 'committee chairmanship' or 'Seventh Day Adventism' as of 'homosexuality'.
>
> (McIntosh 1968)

> My goal has not been to trace the development of 'the lesbian'. There is, of course, no such entity outside of the absurd constructions of textbook and pulp novel writers of the first half of the twentieth century . . . my definition of post-1920s lesbianism [is]: you are a lesbian if you say you are (at least to yourself).
>
> (Faderman 1991)

> 'Lesbian' is a historical construction of comparatively recent date and . . . there is no eternal lesbian essence outside the frame of cultural change and historical determination.
>
> (Fuss 1991)

The somewhat absolutist position proposed by Foucault, that 'the homosexual' as a type of person came into being only as a result of the taxonomic activities of nineteenth-century sexologists, is now recognised as too simplistic. Queer historians have recently presented ample evidence of the social recognition of people we would now call 'lesbian' or 'gay' in seventeenth-century Britain (Donoghue 1993, Norton 1992):

> Lesbians have been badly served by dictionaries, whose authors keep misreading or ignoring our culture. We find that long before the late nineteenth-century publications of the sexologists there was a variety of terms for sexual passion between women, as well as specific labels for the type of woman considered likely to love and have sex with another.
>
> (Donoghue 1993: 7)

Although Foucault's extreme historical constructionist position is untenable, it remains the case that seventeenth-century British 'lesbians' (and Donoghue traces the word 'lesbian' further back than previous scholars) were embedded in a cultural space unimaginably different from that which British culture assigns to contemporary lesbians. The cultural dissonance which the passage of time introduces into the meaning of 'lesbian' is dramatic but probably less so than that associated with place. A seventeenth-century 'lesbian' (and the word must have scare quotes if it is to be tracked across time and space, to reaffirm its inadequacy) living in the Punjab would not have recognised her supposed counterpart in Bejing or Edinburgh. 'Lesbian' is a nexus of meanings which coalesce at the dynamic interface of the body, the self and the social.

The postmodern proliferation of truth-positions and refusal to subscribe to meta-narrative coherence sits with particular ease among this crowd of vanishing lesbians. Not only is the taxonomic vocabulary of sexualities (heterosexual, homosexual, lesbian) a recent invention but, in the coining of the words, the creatures themselves were born. Lillian Faderman is in no doubt that sexologists did not merely *describe* a pre-existing entity – 'the lesbian' – but enabled her to self-define, to organise with others into groups, to exist as a social being and to develop a lesbian subjectivity (Faderman 1981, 1991). Once the social role – the label – is available, it enables individuals to make meaning out of their experiences for themselves and others, meanings which were not possible before. Incorporating such meanings into a lived subjectivity also involves, as we have seen here, a continual evaluative assessment of their felt truth, an on-going process of questioning, challenging, rejecting, replacing, disrupting or embodying the 'lesbian' of various hegemonic or oppositional discourses. Additionally, group solidarity in the face of hostility and stigma tends to reify the semantic categories contested within and between the subordinated group and its oppressors. In a very real sense, 'the lesbian' and 'the lesbian community' are products of oppression.

This is in marked contrast to the construction of *heterosexuality*, whose privileged position as hegemonic norm renders definition or even self-aware *identity* redundant. Thus, heterosexual feminists invited to contribute to a special 'Heterosexuality' issue of *Feminism and Psychology* were almost unanimous in their discomfort with and tendency to reject 'heterosexual' as an ascribed identity:

> Why was anyone so sure? Because I am married? Or because my husband seems 'straight'? Is it about my hairdo or my shoes or the things I have said or not said?[4] . . . How did the heteros get picked out?
>
> (Gergen in Kitzinger and Wilkinson 1993: 62)

Heterosexuality has remained almost totally untheorised and unnamed, precisely because of its staus as norm. The anxiety with which the contributors to the special issue distanced themselves from the label and strove to reassert their specialness, their ontological slipperiness, offers a glimpse into the struggles over naming, privilege and identity from a new and revealing vantage point.

A radical deconstructionist/post-structuralist position insists that 'lesbian' is a sign as amorphous and shifting as any other, bearing at any one time the multiple and contradictory sets of meanings available for encoding in a particular historical/cultural context. The postmodern lesbian is perhaps 'invisible' in an entirely new way, as Catharine Stimpson suggests:

> A 'lesbian identity' once entailed invisibility because no one wanted to see her. Now a 'lesbian identity' might entail invisibility because the lesbian, like some supernatural creature of myth and tale, shows that no identity is stable enough to claim the reassurances of permanent visibility.
>
> (Stimpson 1992)

We seem to have come full circle in the last hundred years, as those temporarily powerful words 'homosexual' and 'heterosexual' are exposed by deconstruction as inadequate and fictitious. Such fictions, of gender and sexuality, have been deployed by and through the discursive practices of superordinate social groups (men, heterosexuals) in order to maintain their dominance over subordinate groups (women, homosexuals). Questions of identity are politically and strategically important, not merely self-indulgent, semantic game-playing. 'Lesbian' must, then, be understood as what Weeks terms a 'necessary fiction'. Lesbians share with gay men the stigmatised existence of the sexual outlaw and with women the oppressed existence of the sexually subordinated.[5] We must not fail to ask in whose interests it is that 'lesbian' be either deconstructed or reified and what strategic interventions are necessary in order to safeguard the interests of those of us who currently call ourselves lesbians and those who may need to do so in future.

THE METAPHORICAL DYKE: TOWARDS A STRATEGIC SEMANTICS OF SEXUALITY

Intellectually, the essentialist position on identity is redundant. Politically, too, the very idea of 'identity', historically and culturally contigent as it is, can prove troublesome, as Freedman *et al.* suggest:

> Such a focus on identity may in fact limit inquiry to those cultures in which lesbian identity and survival *as lesbians* are crucial matters of concern; it may hinder cross-cultural analysis, for example, because it provides inadequate vocabulary for discussion of relationships among Third-World women. . . . Discussion of lesbianism in these terms has relevance only where identity and sexuality are entwined and where personal identity is itself a cultural value.
>
> (Freedman *et al.* 1985)

Yet in order to survive and resist, any marginalised/stigmatised group is obliged to establish at least a rudimentary sense of group identity, or a uniting essence around which to organise. Queerbashers and influential homophobes are not about to modify their behaviour on being told that their aggression is directed against a semantic chimera. Identity politics may appear, from the protected enclaves of the academy, to be intellectually naive and pragmatically divisive, but identity is strategically essential to the struggles of oppressed groups, as feminists and Black women have insisted.

This focussing upon our own oppression is embodied in the concept of identity politics. We believe that the most profound and potentially the most radical politics come directly out of our own identity, as opposed to working to end someone else's oppression.

(Combahee River Collective 1982)

Unless we recognise the interactive nature of what might be thought of as 'identifiction' – the discursive production and allocation of identities through the deployment of which relations of power are maintained and contested – the multiply mediated 'lesbian' positioned across essence/ construct remains embedded in the realm of theory and may not be strategised politically. In many ways, this is analagous to what has become of the word 'woman' in feminist theory and praxis. Julia Kristeva recognises the political Janus-vision which the feminist deconstruction of gender necessitates:

The belief that 'one is a woman' is almost as absurd and obscurantist as the belief that 'one is a man'. I say 'almost' because there are still many goals which women can achieve: freedom of abortion and contraception, day care centres for children, equality on the job etc. Therefore, we must use 'we are women' as an advertisement or slogan for our demands. On a deeper level, however, a woman cannot 'be'; it is something which does not even belong in the order of *being*.

(Kristeva, in Tong 1989)

Strategically, then, a degree of, or moments of, essentialism are necessary. Deconstruction, however important its function to disrupt the continuities of hegemonic discourses, may all too inevitably lead to political paralysis in a world where, after all, the ideological nature of 'oppression' interpenetrates with the material.

'ESSENTIAL' FOR POLITICAL REASONS?

Historically, both sexual politics and the politics of the erotic have coalesced at times around an essentialist position. It is difficult to see how this could have been otherwise, since the subordination of women and the stigmatisation of sexual deviance both depend on the naturalisation of taxonomic practice – the construction of difference as essential. 'Woman' and 'homosexual' are both naturalised and 'made real' within and for the implementation of their excision from the body politic.[6]

The radical feminist response to the essentialist argument that women are intrinsically inferior to men led to the development of apparently contradictory positions. Having moved beyond a liberalism which seeks 'equality' with men within a pre-existing male-identified political and discursive matrix (Grosz 1990a), radical feminists insist variously on the ethical *superiority* of women, or insist on deconstructing sexual difference as a social artefact. The women's peace movement and 'cultural feminism', with its rituals of goddess-worship and the revaluing of the archetypal feminine, are rooted in a feminist essentialism. As such, they offer a very necessary resource for the support and spiritual sustenance of women struggling against patriarchy (Christ 1991). They also offer a powerful challenge to the doctrine of a male supreme being and expose as gendered the relations of power inherent in and sanctified by the monotheistic religions. This interwoven essentialism/deconstruction is important to feminist politics. Its complexity alerts us to the problematic relationship between essence and construct, which may appear to be a diametric opposition but which, in fact, is more of an interactive and dialectic one. There are few political gains to be had from attempting to map a purist deconstructionism on to a social realm organised around essence. Deconstructing masculinity, for example, is not a complete strategy when 'it is not masculinity *per se* which is valorised in our culture but the *masculine male*' (Gatens 1991) (emphasis in original). This logic is even more rigid in the context of sexuality; it is, indeed, not heterosexuality but the heterosexuality of heterosexuals around which the politics of the erotic are structured (anything else being bisexuality and, hence, perverse, or queer or just kinky).

SEIZING THE ESSENTIALIST MOMENT: AIDS AND SECTION 28

Essentialism functions in much the same way for queers as matriarchal religions for feminists. The ability, which a homosexual essence affords, to search the bitterly policed pages of history for our lesbian and gay 'ancestors', gives that validating sense of archival continuity so fundamental to the self-esteem of hounded minorities (Chauncey *et al.* 1989, Vance 1989). It also enables otherwise scattered individuals to organise as groups (Faderman 1991) in response to attacks against them. The struggle against Section 28 of the 1988 Local Government Act in Britain (comparable to the struggle over the Briggs Amendment in the USA) is a good example of the uses to which essentialism tends to be put.

Section 28 is symptomatic of the growth of the New Right, linked to religious fundamentalism (though not to the same degree as in the USA) and promising to 'roll back the state' while at the same time insisting on the state's right and obligation to police intimate behaviour more than at any time since the third Reich (Wilton 1992b). In Britain, the Thatcher government promulgated an ideology of punitive individualism, dismantling the apparatus of the Welfare State in favour of individual self-sufficiency carried to radical extremes, and advocated 'discipline', both fiscal and personal (though not erotically charged, as Operation Spanner shows!), as the solution to the twin evils of permissiveness and recession. Section 28, forbidding the 'promotion' of homosexuality by local authorities, was a response to the successful equal opportunities strategies of the so-called 'loony left' local councils. It was also, for the first time in British Parliamentary history, an attack on homosexual *identities and lifestyles* rather than homosexual acts and was the first Act of Parliament to target lesbians. The reaction of lesbians and gay men and their supporters was to organise around a putative homosexual essence in two main ways.

First there was the argument, familiar from the traditional egalitarian stance of the early homophile organisations (Faderman 1991), that you cannot 'promote' homosexuality. We are born this way, runs the argument, this is not a disease you can catch nor a habit you can be lured into. If homosexuality is innate it is demonstrably unjust to penalise homosexuals for something they cannot help. These arguments were vigorously rehearsed in Parliamentary debates on Section 28.

> I do not believe that it is possible to make a heterosexual into a homosexual. . . . It is not a disease to be caught and it cannot be taught. . . . All the evidence suggests that for 99.9 per cent of the population over the age of seven or eight, homosexuality is determined.
> (Allan Roberts, Labour MP, in Roelofs 1991)

> Encouraging people to be homosexual . . . is an absurd notion in any case. We are what we are. It is impossible to force or encourage someone into a different sexuality from that which pertains to them.
> (Chris Smith, out gay Labour MP, ibid.)

While this retreat into essentialism was derided by a vocal section of the lesbian and gay community (Roelofs 1991), it was a direct reponse to the whole spirit of Section 28, which is predicated upon a non-essentialist model of homosexuality precisely as something which may be learned, taught or 'promoted'. US anti-gay campaigner Anita Bryant insists that 'homosexuals cannot reproduce, so they have to recruit our children'. If homosexuality was so biologically determined as to prevent homosexuals reproducing then it would not be possible to 'recruit' heterosexuals into homosexuality. The rhetoric of homophobia has always been an ill informed mix of essentialist and anti-essentialist, speaking of homo-sexuality as a disease, a contamination, an abomination or a personal weakness to be striven against by moral crusade and rigorous self-discipline. It is hard to devise an intellectually coherent challenge to a position so lacking in logic or rationality.

The second strategic use made of essentialism in the fight against Section 28 was the rallying call to lesbians and gay men to unite on the basis of a shared homosexual identity. This, too, is a strategy with a long history in the twentieth-century struggles for homosexual rights: 'Activists not only had to mobilize a constituency; first they had to create one' (d'Emilio 1983). Such a constituency is, by definition, organised around the belief that the political agendas of lesbians and of gay men are best served by agreement to self-define as members of one group, 'homosexuals', 'gay people' or 'queers'. In the face of legislation which clearly made the assumption of a unifying gender-neutral homo-sexuality, the choice was to organise around that homosexuality rather than disrupting it by presenting pluralities of gender/desire. This strategy was not without its critics:

> The Clause . . . was not attacking homosexual desire, the existence of which it basically accepted, but lesbian and gay *identity*, the public expression of which it believed was morally wrong. What we needed to do in response was to defend lesbian and gay identities as *choices*, responsible, healthy, life-enhancing choices. Instead we took up an essentially apologist position ('We're sorry, but we can't help it').
>
> (Hamer *et al.* 1991)

There appears to be a link, tentatively marked throughout lesbian and gay political history, between oppression/danger and expressed essentialism. Indeed, Diana Fuss goes further, suggesting that the degree to which essentialism is present within sub-cultural discourse correlates with the degree of oppression felt, something which is clearly different for lesbians and for gay men.

> If the adherence to essentialism is a measure of the degree to which a particular political group has been culturally oppressed . . . then the stronger lesbian endorsement of identity and identity politics may well indicate that lesbians inhabit a more precarious and less secure position than gay men.
>
> (Fuss 1989)

The material and ideological realities of male power necessarily result in lesbians 'inhabiting a more precarious position' than gay men. They also delineate the parameters of specifically *sexual* (as opposed to erotic)[7] power relations among queers. From the early days of the homophile Mattachine Society in the USA, 'male homosexuals defined gayness in terms that negated the experience of lesbians and conspired to keep them out' (d'Emilio 1983). Gay men may or may not choose to critique the social ascription and policing of gender roles in relation to male sexual behaviour – very few of them have articulated a sexual–political critique of any sophistication. Thomas Yingling is among the handful of gay men who recognise that 'lesbians – as women – are marked in our culture in such a way that their "difference" is inescapable; gay men, on the other hand, are marked in a different way that does not preclude their "passing" or their negotiations of many of the privileges of masculinity even if known to be gay' (Yingling 1991). Small wonder then that lesbian identity – lesbian 'essence' – is so vigorously endorsed by many lesbians.

A cynical reading suggests that lesbians fulfil the role of some kind of political 'reserve army of labour' within feminism and within queer activism, to be called up when needed and otherwise ignored. It is probably more truthful to recognise that, as 'lesbian' is a negotiated subject position in more or less constant flux, so it is obliged to perform *reactively* in response to its strategic deployment *by others* in a multitude of discourses. For example, recognising that the homophobia which, like some malign apocalyptic horseman, straddles the back of the HIV/AIDS epidemic does not bother with niceties of gender, lesbians have aligned themselves with gay men in the AIDS field. '[T]he two terms "lesbian" and "gay", driven apart by rapidly accelerating differences in visibility and privilege marking them through the supposed halcyon days of the 70s, have been brought together in (AIDS) discourse' (Yingling 1991). Far from being the result of gay men enlisting lesbians in the battle (on the contrary, lesbians are conspicuously absent from the overwhelming bulk of gay men's writing about AIDS), lesbian involvement sprang from their willingness to align themselves politically with gay men against homophobia.

CONCLUSION

Amid all this clamorous contestation we must surely abandon as misguided the attempt at a straightforward lexicographical definition of 'lesbian'. Yet we must not betray the flesh and bone which inhabits and enacts the lesbian body and lesbian desire. Lesbians occupy a position which is at the same time both fragile and dangerous and which is a uniquely powerful and paradigmatically disruptive site eccentric to the heteropolar signifying economy:

> The homo in relation to the hetero, much like the feminine in relation to the masculine, operates as an indispensible interior exclusion – an outside which is inside interiority making the articulation of the latter possible, a transgression of the border which is necessary to constitute the border as such.
>
> > (Fuss 1991)

But lesbians transgress *both* sets of borders and, as such, as the subordinate in the (gender/erotic) heterobinary, are constructed as doubly 'other' and repudiated as such. Lesbian may well be a social construct, but no alternative, extra-social, extra-discursive mode of les-being is possible. The queer community merely reinforces and re-enacts women's subordination to men in a specific, sub-cultural context, while the feminist deconstruction of lesbian identity as a continuum of experience common to *all* women threatens to deny the lived experience of lesbian women, as Sheila Jeffreys warns:

> Women who simply have 'best friends' who are women share neither lesbian oppression nor lesbian experience. So long as we keep the definition of lesbianism open enough to include heterosexual women who love their women friends, it will be hard to articulate what is specific about the experience and oppression of lesbians and to develop the strength to fight compulsory heterosexuality and the invisibility of lesbians.
>
> > (Jeffreys 1989)

Additionally, deconstruction may serve to reinforce not only sexism but racism as well as this anonymous Black lesbian makes clear:

> Torn between the homophobia of the black community and the racism of the white lesbian movement, I need, as a black lesbian, to speak for myself and in my own voice, which is not the voice of the white world. I do not want my black experience filtered through your white academic language.
>
> > (Kitzinger 1987)

Deconstructing 'lesbianism' or 'race' does make visible the discursive mechanisms of social control. But it does not abolish material reality for lesbians deprived of housing, employment, their children or their liberty *because of their lesbianism* or for the majority of Black people humiliated and impoverished in the interests of white people around the world *because of their blackness*.

Caught at the dynamic confluence of feminist and queer theory but inadequately incorporated within either; exposed as the demonised chimera of the patriarchal imagination but inadequately protected by poststructuralism from the sticks, stones and prisons of heteropatriarchal materiality; lesbian women and the metaphorical 'lesbian' co-exist in unease. Perhaps it is more appropriate to understand lesbian-ness as activity rather than entity, 'les-being' rather than 'lesbian'. What is certain is that the politics of naming is at the heart of lesbian studies. It is not so much 'the lesbian' which we study, as the multiple, shifting processes which the lesbian body inhabits and enacts at the permeable meniscus between the social and the self.

NOTES

1 Well, how would *you* fancy a spot of 'partner manipulation'? And what the hell is it anyway? Another example of how embarrassed euphemism destroys any credibility for lesbian sex . . .
2 Storr is basing this statement on such inadequate information about lesbians that he seems unaware of the substantial numbers of women who (even at the time this was written) choose lesbianism after years of heterosexuality or who leave marriages for lesbian partnerships.
3 There is some disagreement about what Ti-Grace Atkinson intended by her now famous statement. Lesbians who were there at the time remember her suggesting that because feminism was a *theory* and lesbianism was a *practice*, there was no way in which lesbianism could be seen as analogous to, or implicit in, feminism (see p. 93). However, it has been adopted as a lesbian slogan to mean precisely the opposite.
4 Well yes . . . probably all those.
5 By 'sexually subordinated' I mean that women are materially and ideologically subordinate to men both on the grounds of sexual difference (in Freudian/Lacanian terms by being excluded *because of* their lack of a penis from the economy of significance, which is phallogocentrism) and *by means of* sexual difference (rape and sexual violence being deployed, as radical feminists suggest, in order to maintain men's power over women).
6 It is undoubtedly true that the ideological justification/motivation for the political disenfranchisement of women and homosexuals (of both sexes) is inter-related, something which will be discussed in Chapter 4.
7 Semantics are problematic here! I am using 'sexual' in this instance to refer to physiological sex (whether a person is 'male' or 'female') rather than gender, which is generally understood, at least within the lesbian and gay milieu, to be a social category with a certain mutability. 'Erotic' refers to the realm of desire and fulfilment.

Chapter 3

Invisible and erased
Uses and abuses of history

> [A]mong the tribes there were women warriors, women leaders, women shamans, women husbands, but whether any of these were lesbians is seldom mentioned.
>
> (Allen 1989)

The tools and conditions of oppression are not solely material, rather the materialities of oppression are both reflected in and reproduced/ reinforced by the ideological, which itself both informs and is deployed through the cultural. Complex dynamics are at work among politics, history, subjectivity and representation. History is not an objective narrative, recounting past events as they 'really were', any more than current representational practices simply mirror a pre-existing contemporary reality. In a profoundly logocentric culture such as ours there is a constant process of struggle and negotiation to determine whose words are heard and whose are silenced, whose thoughts are recorded and whose erased from the record, whose truth gets told and whose denied. The datasphere is a battleground; libraries are wars in progress. Within the postmodern paradigm 'truth' is no longer understood as an absolute but as the (temporary, local) credibility of specific discourses among competing miriads. We may not understand ourselves as uncovering or laying bare extra-textual 'reality' but as constructing or reconstructing necessarily contingent, partial and plural narratives. Lesbian history will not be able to discover the truth about lesbians, for no such truth exists. Does this mean that we are left with nothing more than an infinitely diminishing present moment, that 'lesbian' is just a momentary interference pattern in time and space? Yes, but in this it is no different from any other human being, from 'proletariat' or 'courtesan' to 'scientist' or 'peasant'. All history is a *retrospective* meaning-making: living individuals did not think of themselves as 'hunter-gatherer nomads' or 'pre-capitalist agrarian labourers'.

The narrative content of history is of secondary importance to lesbian studies. More significant is the politics of history-making, the questions of whose interests are best served by the construction of certain historical narratives and the uses to which such narratives are put. In this chapter I want to examine the ways in which historical strategies of writing (constructing a lesbian history, recording lesbian biographies/ autobiographies, redefining certain significant individuals as lesbian, etc.) may be deployed against strategies of erasure (denying lesbian history, suppressing evidence of eroticism between women, 'rescuing' significant individuals from the charge of lesbianism, etc.).

HISTORIES: IDENTITIES

Historical inquiry has a crucial part to play in the strategies of decon-struction. It exposes, for example, the constructedness of taxonomic fictions such as 'race'. Embedded as we are in the ideology of a racist culture, it is a shock to learn that dark skin colour has not always represented to whites the stigmatising signifier of inferiority which it is today. That information reveals that racism is a social institution with a political history (see, for example, Ware 1992). A position informed by this history enables us to problematise racism rather than race and to denaturalise racism as constructed and contingent (and hence expose its deployment as political) rather than as the 'natural' individual/ psychological reponse to the unfamiliar.

An historical perspective clearly has specific and important benefits to offer lesbians and lesbian studies. It enables us to problematise heterosexism, by recognising its historical shifts as indicative of its political nature rather than seeing it as a universal or transcendent psychological, and hence unchangeable, entity (Kitzinger 1987). Lesbian historical scholarship may take the following forms:

- celebrating lesbian groups or individuals who have 'left their mark on history';
- identifying the mechanisms of erasure whereby lesbian existence has been deleted from the record;
- constructing a history of the idea 'lesbian' and its deployment;
- recording accounts of lesbian and gay movement politics;
- devising strategies to resist the on-going erasure of lesbians from the record.

Each of these will be discussed here, focusing on the strategic import-. ance of an affirmative historicity for lesbian studies and for lesbians.

SAPPHO, GLUCK AND LET'S CLAIM VIRGINIA – GREAT DYKES OF HERSTORY

If 'lesbian' is a contested and evanescent product of cultural negotiation rather than a sub-species of human being, what sense does it make to speak of the great lesbians of history? Strictly speaking, none at all, as lesbian scholars generally agree (Faderman 1991, Vance 1989). Indeed:

> [g]iven a strict anti-essentialist or social constructionist perspective, we cannot use 'lesbian' to refer to any identity or behaviour pre-dating the late nineteenth century, and may need to restrict our inquiries to Western capitalist societies.
>
> (Zimmerman 1992a)

Yet this is to negate the historical enterprise in its entirety, since all other historic-taxonomic classifications are as much products of social and cultural construction as 'lesbian'. It is only because 'lesbian' is such a polyvocally contested construct *today* that its semantic fragility is so brutally apparent when regarded historically. And it is only because the dominant historical narratives of our time (like the dominant 'scientific' narratives) intersect with the hegemonic world-view of the white, male ruling class that they may call themselves truth. As Linda Gordon, commenting on feminist historical scholarship, writes:

> In attempting to reconstruct history, feminists do no more and no less than many groups battling for political power have done before. . . . From the classical world to Tudor England to the Reagan administration, ideologues write and rewrite histories of their imperialisms, successions, and legitimacy, with an eye to raising money for armies.
>
> (Gordon 1991)

History is a story told for a present purpose and hence is intrinsically mythologising. The tendency among lesbians to mythologise lesbian 'foremothers' is often naive but it is no more or less bad history than the mythologising of figures such as Winston Churchill, Abraham Lincoln or John F. Kennedy. Casting a lesbian eye over some great dykes of the past can reveal the mechanisms of heterosexist suppression as well as offering a sense of continuity through time.

Was Sappho a sapphist?

Very little is known about Sappho, and there is considerable controversy over whether she herself was a lesbian or not. Many critics, motivated by a throroughly modern heterosexism, have felt the need to rescue this important lyric poet of antiquity from the accusation of unnatural love. Typical of these is Sappho 'expert' David Robinson, who wrote that it was simply not possible for a poet of Sappho's sensitivity to be a lesbian:

> It is against the nature of things that a woman who has given herself up to unnatural and inordinate practices which defy the moral instinct and throw the soul into disorder, practices which harden and petrify the soul, should be able to write in perfect obedience to the laws of vocal harmony, imaginative portrayal, and arrangement of the details of thought. The nature of things does not admit of such an inconsistency. Sappho's love for flowers, moreover, afford another luminous testimony. A bad woman as well as a pure woman might love roses, but a bad woman does not love the small and hidden wild flowers of the field . . . as Sappho did.
>
> (Robinson 1963, in Klaich 1985)

That such gross irrationality should be acceptable within academic discourse as recently as the 1960s is testimony to the totality with which the pathological model of lesbianism infiltrated Western culture. It is not only those motivated by loathing, however, who reject 'lesbian' as an accurate or appropriate label for the great poet.[1] Among historians 'the great Sappho question', as André Lardinois terms it, remains precisely whether or not she was, in the erotic sense, a lesbian. Lardinois himself, suggesting that Sappho's erotic relationships with young women took the form of institutionalised initiation rituals, is in no doubt what the answer is:

> We may conclude that in the case of Sappho we are dealing at the most with short relationships between an adult woman and a young, marriageable girl. To call these relationships 'lesbian' is anachronistic. Whether the word applies to Sappho herself, her inner life, is impossible to assess. Actually it constitutes a nonsensical question. Even if, by modern standards Sappho were to be considered lesbian, her experience must have been very different, living as she did in a different age with different notions and different types of sexuality.
>
> (Lardinois 1989)

So what *do* we know about the eponymous sapphist? Tantalisingly little, as befits the metaphorical ancestress of such a fluid community. She lived *c.* 612–558 BC, and was a renowned poet in her own lifetime, to the extent that statues were erected to honour her and coins – some of which were collected by Renee Vivien during her pilgrimage to Lesbos with Natalie Barney (Livia 1993) – struck bearing her portrait: 'No woman of her time was more celebrated' (Klaich 1985). Socrates and Plato were both fulsome in her praise, Plato naming her the tenth Muse. She performed some kind of leadership/teacher function to a group of girls and young women from wealthy families and appears to have run some sort of establishment for them on Lesbos, one of the larger Aegean islands.

Her writings, which were proclaimed as the zenith of the poetic arts in her lifetime, have suffered extensively from the ravages of social upheaval through the centuries. They were publicly burned in the Christian attempt to suppress paganism in the Eastern Roman Empire *c.* AD 380, and again by Pope (later Saint) Gregory VII (1073–1085) in Rome, along with many other ancient writings. It was not until the early Renaissance that Sappho was rediscovered, in the frustrating form of quoted extracts in classical Greek and Latin texts, by Italian scholars fired by the enthusiasm for the classical pagan world which fuelled the Renaissance.

Translated into English, the fragments (only one or two entire poems were found) were forcibly reshaped to construct a heterosexual Sappho, a misreading which went unchallenged until two Oxford University scholars excavated an ancient rubbish heap at Oxyrhynchus (now called Behneseh) in Egypt and unearthed, among other marvels, discarded papyrus scrolls of Sappho's verse. The scrolls were all that remained of pagan libraries, trashed in favour of Christian literature, and had been torn into strips before being consigned to the scrap heap, but enough had been preserved in the dry Egyptian climate to dispel the myth of an unproblematically heterosexual Sappho. Many were unambiguously erotic and clearly addressed to women.

Ruthlessly scattered by historical events, the few remaining fragments of her poetry construct a kind of join-the-dots puzzle, an outline open enough for those who wish to fill it in with details of their own. She is paradigmatic of the constitutive processes of history – with so little evidence of the 'real' woman, the mechanisms whereby everyone can construct their own Sappho are clear to see – none of which detracts from her iconographic and metaphorical importance in a lesbian context. It is exciting enough that a woman writer held such a lofty position; that she should have been a lesbian (however we may understand that term as applied to a woman who lived two and a half thousand years ago) makes her a powerful totem indeed.

Nearer home: famous lesbians of more recent times

Women have undoubtedly been having sex with each other throughout history, although it is unlikely that the socio-cultural meanings of their behaviours are amenable to retrospective comprehension. Of course, one major problem is that the vast majority of individuals leave no trace in the record. Unless a woman came into the sphere of a record-keeping institution (such as a convent or court of law), or became celebrated in her own time, we have no way of knowing that she existed. It is possible to investigate general social attitudes to sex between women from sources such as court records, ecclesiastical pronouncements and scandalous reports of the behaviour of nuns or the aristocracy (such as the charge of lesbianism popularly levelled at Marie Antoinette). However, the interpretation of such sources is problematic: they were generally inspired at the time by a political or religious agenda and reading them through the haze of modern ideas about sexuality and intimacy loads them with another set of assumptions.

To disentangle the struggles over 'lesbian history', it is easier to focus on public figures who lived at a time when love and eroticism between women was open to interpretation within the sexological paradigm, when it was possible to live a lesbian life more or less as a lesbian living in the West today would understand it. Among the better known of such women are Rosa Bonheur, Dame Ethyl Smyth, Gertrude Stein, Radclyffe Hall and Gluck.

Rosa Bonheur (1822–99) was a French painter, thought by many to be the best painter of her generation. She was awarded the Croix de la Legion d'Honneur in 1864 by the Empress Eugenie, then Regent of France. It was the first time the Croix had been awarded by a woman to a woman, and the Empress 'had wished that the last act of my regency be dedicated to showing that in my eyes genius has no sex ' (Petersen and Wilson 1976). Bonheur was unique among her generation and her class in her insistence on wearing men's clothes. Crossdressing was illegal, so she was obliged to carry a certificate signed by the prefect of police giving her official permission to do so. Her justification was that for France's greatest animal painter to wear long, trailing skirts to sketch in slaughter houses and cattle markets as she did was impractical. This was undoubtedly true. However, biographers suggest that Bonheur was a product of her time in subscribing to the mythos of genius as masculine and acted out her own genius accordingly (Faderman 1981, Greer 1979).

As a 'male-identified' genius, she was able to achieve what she did thanks to the dedication and love of the woman who fulfilled the traditional role of genius' wife, Nathalie Micas. The two women lived together until Micas' death in 1875, after which Bonheur fell into a deep and unproductive depression until the arrival of an American artist, Anna Klumpke, who gave up her own career to live with Rosa for the last months of her life, and who subsequently wrote her biography (Greer 1979, Heller 1987).

Surely Bonheur belongs unquestionably in lesbian history? Yet commentators disagree about whether or not she may be called a lesbian. Petersen and Wilson (1976) insist on the 'purity' of her relationships with Micas and Klumpke.[2] Greer (1979) remains uncommitted about her lesbianism, reflecting on the possibility that the relationship with Micas was 'not carnal' and that 'however much sex there was in their relationship, there was no dearth of love', while Faderman (1981) accepts that Bonheur and Micas were lesbians. For Dell Richards (1990) Bonheur is both a lesbian and a feminist.

Such controversy is clearly motivated by the commentator's own conflicting positions on lesbianism. It is unsurprising that those authors unquestioningly content to call Bonheur a lesbian are themselves lesbians. Different strategies of denial must be employed when confronted with 'out' lesbians such as Dame Ethyl Smyth.

Ethyl Smyth (1858–1944), classical composer and Suffragist, is one important English lesbian still awaiting a detailed feminist or lesbian biography. Honoured and revered in her time – she was made a Dame in 1922 – her works were performed widely and a public festival was held to honour her on the occasion of her seventy-fifth birthday. It was she who composed the 'March of the Women' for the Suffragette movement. Yet the British loved her as a character rather than as a serious composer, and it was in Germany and by non-British fellow composers (Tchaikovsky, Brahms, Mahler and Grieg) that she was taken most seriously as a musician. She herself said:

Because I have conducted my own operas and love sheepdogs; because I generally dress in tweeds, and sometimes. . . have even conducted in them; because I was a militant Suffragette and seized the chance of beating time to [my] March of the Women from the window of my cell in Holloway prison with a toothbrush; because I

have written books, spoken speeches, broadcast and don't always
make sure that my hat is on straight . . . I am well known.

(Smyth/Crichton 1990)

Photographs taken of Smyth at the turn of the century show a dapper
figure in masculine attire, hat at a rakish angle. She is remembered (and
trivialised) as the Battling Dame of British Music, a comment on the
unacceptably unfeminine qualities of her music. Archbishop Benson is
said to have remarked acidly of her Mass that God was not implored but
commanded to have mercy. Unremarkably, her lesbianism is not mentioned in her entry in the *Oxford Companion to Music* (Scholes 1969),
but then, neither is Tchaikovsky's homosexuality. Smyth has simply
been 'forgotten'. Although she lived well into the twentieth century, her
work is now seldom performed and she was recently 'rediscovered' by
the 1994 Henry Wood Promenade concerts in London.

Smyth was characteristically forthright about her love affairs with
women, making it impossible for homophobic biographers to claim
heterosexuality for her. Without such personal testimony, even the most
celebrated lesbian is liable to be 'straightened out' by those determined
to protect the great from the taint of perversion, as the case of Gertrude
Stein shows.

Gertrude Stein (1874–1946), is one of the giants of twentieth-century
experimental literature. Perhaps only James Joyce is of comparable
stature. Her life-long 'marriage' with Alice Toklas must be one of the
most (in)famous lesbian partnerships ever. Yet, as recently as 1971,
'Patricia Meyerowitz wrote that Gertrude Stein and Alice B. Toklas
were only friends. They made a home together and had an emotional
bond that held them together, she admitted, but "lesbians never"'
(Richards 1990). This, in spite of the well-known fact that Stein's
oeuvre includes some of the most graphically erotic (albeit coded)
writing in the history of literature, addressed to Toklas:

Tiny dish of delicious which
Is my wife and all
And a perfect ball

(Stein, in Souhami 1991)

Gertrude and Alice became legendary. Feted as a couple they were
photographed by Cecil Beaton, Alfred Stieglitz and Man Ray and were
friends with Picasso, Hemingway, Matisse and Scott Fitzgerald. They
were at the centre of the modernist bohemian artistic world which

flourished so dazzlingly in Europe and the United States up until the Second World War, and became wealthy on the proceeds of Stein's literary success (Souhami 1991). Gertrude's achievement makes her arguably the most 'establishment' lesbian since Sappho, though the experimental nature of her writing (where 'cows' and 'caesar' become sexual code-words) does not endear her to a wide lesbian audience. Popularity among lesbians is reserved for a far lesser writer, Radclyffe Hall.

Radclyffe Hall (1883–1943), christened Marguerite and known as John for most of her adult life, has become notorious as the writer who penned *The Well of Loneliness*, the first novel in the English language to openly plead the cause of lesbians. *The Well* roused the ire of the heterosexual establishment. James Dougles wrote in the *Sunday Express*: 'I would rather give a healthy boy or girl a phial of prussic acid than this novel', and suggested that it would 'destroy Christianity' (19 August 1928). The publisher was prosecuted for obscenity within six weeks and flocks of celebrities lined up to defend the book, including Virginia and Leonard Woolf, E. M. Forster, Julian Huxley and Vita Sackville-West, none of whom was allowed by the court to testify. Yet it was not wholeheartedly endorsed by contemporary lesbians. Romaine Brooks, an openly lesbian painter, called it a 'ridiculous, trite, superficial book' and Violet Trefusis, Vita Sackville-West's lover, thought it 'loathsome' (Richards 1990). Feminist and critical opinion remain divided on its political and literary merit (O'Rourke 1989, Ruehl 1982), its radicalism as an anti-homophobic treatise (Ruehl 1982, Stimpson 1981) and the significance of its author's Catholicism (Glasgow 1992).

The Well provoked the first major public debate in Britain and the United States about the nature and significance of lesbian-ness and, in so doing, ensured that the sexological construct of the 'invert' entered popular consciousness. Hall subscribed to Havelock Ellis' idea of the invert as a member of the third sex, biologically and psychologically distinct from both men and women. She persuaded Ellis to write a foreword to the book, believing that once the world understood that lesbianism was congenital, natural justice would overcome prejudice and bigotry. For her, God made the invert as deliberately as he made the giraffe or hedgehog. Inadequate and apologistic as this position seems to us now, at the time it represented for many lesbians the only way out of a maze of guilt, shame and self-loathing (Faderman 1981, O'Rourke 1989).

The Well of Loneliness remains the most well-known lesbian novel. It has been called 'The Lesbian Bible' (Martin and Lyon 1972). The mini-industry of cultural and academic production concerning *The Well* is precisely *because* of its significance in the social history of sexuality; most of Radclyffe Hall's other novels are almost completely unknown and uncriticised. The notoriety of *The Well* and its trial have ensured that Hall cannot be subject to the kind of retrospective 'straightening' that homophobic critics attempt for Stein. The sheer amount of documentary evidence also makes it relatively difficult to 'forget' about her, although there is no doubt that it is thanks to feminist publishers Virago and to lesbian academic commentary that this has not happened. In stark contrast is the vanishing trick played on her no less successful contemporary, Gluck.

Gluck (1895–1978) was born Hannah Gluckstein, but insisted on the unadorned monosyllable all her adult life, although she was called 'Peter' by friends and lovers. She was a painter, who achieved some degree of establishment success and was frequently commissioned to paint official portraits of judges, magistrates, etc. She was an official war artist, and her exhibitions were fashionable events attended on one occasion by Queen Mary. She was something of a society figure: *Homes and Gardens* ran a three-page article on her house and her studio in July 1935 and her remarkable flower paintings were received with far more critical acclaim than the 'masculine strength' of her portraiture, land-scapes or still lives (Souhami 1988). She lived quite openly as a lesbian, dressed in tailored men's clothes, and was passionately involved with a succession of women lovers. Her longest relationship was with Nesta Obermer, whom she painted alongside her own self-portrait in 'Medallion', probably her only well-known work now (it adorns the cover of the Virago edition of *The Well of Loneliness*) and called by Gluck the 'YouWe picture'. She called Nesta 'My own darling wife . . . my divine sweetheart, my love, my life'.

Gluck's was a productive life – she continued painting until the illnesses of her old age prevented her, and her late paintings are masterly. She had a succesful exhibition at the Fine Arts Society in 1973. She worked slowly and meticulously, sometimes taking years to finish one painting, and was obsessive about the quality of the paints she used. She campaigned vigorously to get paint manufacturers to improve the quality of their colours, and Rowney provided her free of charge with specially hand-made paints, ground from lapis lazuli, vermilion and viridian. Her ivory black was made for her in India, using elephant ivory rather than the bone used in commercial paints. It is some indication of her stature that her outrageous perfectionism was catered for in this way!

Yet Gluck is almost invisible within feminist art history, and even within lesbian affirmative scholarship. You may search in vain in the index of key texts (Petersen and Wilson's *Women Artists*, Heller's *Women Artists: An Illustrated History*, Faderman's *Surpassing the Love of Men*) for her name, while Greer allocates just six lines to her in *The Obstacle Race*, suggesting that 'her cross-dressing was part of her intense virginal fastidiousness' and ignoring her lesbianism entirely. Even Richards (1990) includes her under 'Women who wore Men's Clothing' rather than under 'Lesbian Artists'. Were it not for Diana Souhami's (1988) biography, Gluck would have been erased from the record as completely as if she had never lived.

INVISIBLE OR DELETED? CHALLENGING MECHANISMS OF LESBIAN ERASURE

Homosexuality is purged from the pages of history as a matter of course. Gay men's sexuality is subject to denial, obliteration, silence. Yet their erasure is not as total as that to which the lesbian historical subject has been treated. Not only is same-sex eroticism silenced by the narratives of history, but those narratives (together with religion, science, art and philosophy) have been told by men for men and about men. Gay men's sexuality may be left out of the account but lesbians are struck off altogether, our very existence denied. Although we are not told that W. H. Auden, Maynard Keynes, Cecil Beaton, Michelangelo, Cecil Rhodes or Tchaikovsky were homosexual, we have been taught to venerate their accomplishments. The scholar of lesbian history is faced with two problematic sets of dispersal: the destruction of evidence of sexual deviance which dogs any attempt to reclaim a homosexual subject and the tendency of historians simply to ignore women.

The obliteration of women takes two forms. First, a refusal to accept excellence, achievement or ability in women, suppressing any evidence which contradicts women's positioning as inferior to men. The very existence of women novelists, playwrights, inventors, scientists, mathematicians, healers, painters, sculptors, poets or leaders has had to be painstakingly reclaimed (Alic 1986, Greer 1979, Heller 1987, Petersen and Wilson 1976, Spender 1982, Vare and Ptacek 1987, Weidner *et al.* 1988). Second, women as a class have been ignored. Events which concern primarily women, such as the three centuries of European witch-burning during which an estimated nine million women were slaughtered (Daly 1979), or the activism of the Suffragists (MacKenzie 1975/88) are belittled, mocked or passed over with a sentence or two by history books.

This suppression is not unitary but multiple, predicated upon the political imperative to justify and maintain the subordination not only of women but also of working-class people and people of colour. Individual women who have escaped erasure have almost always been able to do so because of their racial privilege and socio-economic status. It is no accident that Bonheur, Smyth, Stein, Radclyffe-Hall and Gluck were all middle-class or aristocratic white women. Class and race privilege may mitigate gender disprivilege, enabling a few women to devote their lives to something other than marriage and domestic labour. It is clear that what we call 'history' privileges the stories of this materially powerful few, relegating working-class women to the generic status of peasant, slave, prostitute or factory hand. Third World women are assumed not to have any pre-colonial history at all.

One of the most important feminist projects has been, therefore, to research and record the lives of Black, lesbian and working-class women and to record the life stories of living women whose voices would otherwise be silenced (Webster 1992, Wilson 1978). While the lesbian-ness of historical figures may be denied and the lesbian-ness of their work erased where possible, being a lesbian does not *per se* prevent women from making their living by writing, painting or composing in the way that being Black or working class – or simply female to begin with – clearly may.

There has been a small explosion recently of cheap, readily available books documenting recent or contemporary lesbian lives. Some are individual autobiographies (Lorde 1982, Manning 1987, Nestle 1987), some biographies (Souhami 1988, 1991), but the majority have been collections of the stories of 'ordinary' lesbians, many recorded in the established tradition of oral history. Their titles often bear witness to the erasure they are challenging – *Invisible Lives* (Barrett 1990), *We Are Everywhere* (Alpert 1988), *Inventing Ourselves* (Hall Carpenter Archives Oral History Group 1989), *Testimonies* (Holmes 1988), *Not A Passing Phase* (Lesbian History Group 1989), *What a Lesbian Looks Like* (National Lesbian and Gay survey 1992), *Finding the Lesbians* (Penelope and Valentine 1990) – and there is a concern, informed by recent feminist praxis, to reflect diversity, to make space for the stories of minority women, older women, disabled women, and to listen to what women in other cultures have to say about their experiences of being lesbian. There are specialist collections of the stories of Jewish women (Beck 1982), older women (Neild and Pearson 1992), women with children (Alpert 1988) and children of lesbian mothers (Rafkin 1990).

Allied to the politically subversive activity of recording lesbian lives is the need to explore and celebrate different ways of being lesbian. A common theme in lesbian coming-out stories is that of individuals deciding that they couldn't possibly be a lesbian because they were not what the books available said lesbians were; men trapped in women's bodies, sick, psychotic, sinful, obsessed with sex or driven by the urge to smoke cigars and wear trousers. Accessible evidence of a plurality of lesbianisms is valuable to those restricted not only by the damning stereotypes of heterosexual prejudice but also by what may be the equally restrictive dictates of fragile lesbian sub-cultures.

ANOTHER ERASURE

Within a marginalised and often ghettoised community, a narrow, normative ethic may be rigorously policed in an anxiety to survive intact in a hostile majority culture. As Plummer notes, 'the [gay] liberationists themselves have started to become key definers of a homosexual role and hence ironically have started to become their own source of regulation' (Plummer 1981a). In a beleaguered milieu, where gender and the erotic are self-consciously recognised as political constructs and where the signifiers of dress codes, hairstyle, etc. are deployed in the interests of establishing and perpetuating an oppositional sartorial discourse, 'private' matters such as fashion, sexual behaviour or the choice to have children can take on an importance *for the community* as well as for the individual. This can result in whole sub-cultural groups or behaviours being marginalised within an already existing marginality, a distressing experience for the women involved.

Thus, lesbians whose presented persona is informed by a public endorsement of sadomasochistic sex are currently demonised by anti-SM lesbians, who see SM as celebrating the dominance/submission dichotomy characteristic of heterosexuality, and some lesbian communities have become polarised around vanilla/SM loyalties. Similarly, the row over whether or not to permit lesbian mothers to bring their boy children to women-only events served to further exclude lesbian mothers – an already vulnerable and isolated group – from the 'community'.

The important conclusion to draw from such internal politicking is that lesbian historical scholarship is no more immune than any other from partiality. There is no unitary lesbian perspective, no monolithic lesbian ethic which makes lesbian history-telling more intrinsically truthful than any other. Butch/femme role playing, for example, around which an entire lesbian community was organised in the 1940s and

1950s in the United States and parts of Europe (Faderman 1991, Nestle 1987, Weeks 1977/90), has been castigated by some lesbian feminists as mere mimicry of heterosexuality (Jeffreys 1989) and hence ignored as part of lesbian cultural history, while other commentators see it as both a necessary strategy for collective survival and an important challenge to gender stereotypes (see essays by Cordova, Kennedy and Davis in Nestle 1992).

I have suggested that reclaiming the lives of individual lesbians is important in order to challenge the discursive mechanisms of erasure by which lesbian possibility is denied and to construct an alternative and oppositional cultural paradigm within which contemporary women may negotiate the meanings of their lesbianism. It is also important to understand the history of lesbians as a group, of lesbianism as a social phenomenon, and of the struggles for lesbian civil and human rights.

SOCIAL CONSTRUCTS FIGHT BACK

Studying sexuality has only relatively recently been accepted as a valid academic enterprise, and homosexuality has only been deemed an appropriate field of scholarship since the early 1970s. Homosexuality has been studied, along with prostitution and other sex-related behaviours problematic within a heterosexist Judaeo-Christian paradigm, precisely because of its deviant status (Hobson 1987, Wells 1982). We have yet to develop a scholarship of heterosexuality (Kitzinger *et al.* 1993, Richardson 1995). Historians of homosexuality have been by and large historians of the *relationship* between homosexuality and heterosexuality, the development of a lesbian or gay male identity and/or sub-culture (d'Emilio 1983, Faderman 1981, 1991, Katz 1983, Weeks 1977/90, 1985 and many essays in Duberman *et al.* 1991), the shifting meanings of the words 'homosexual' and 'lesbian' and, more recently, the history of the lesbian and gay *movement* as a changing set of social and political groupings (Abbott and Love 1972, Blumenfeld and Raymond 1988, Cant and Hemmings 1988, Cruikshank 1992, d'Emilio 1983, Kaufmann and Lincoln 1991, Shepherd 1989).

Historical accounts of recent community struggles and figures are not without problems. It is essential for any oppressed group to be able to chart the ebb and flow of its political standing, to reckon their out and out enemies, to judge the limits of radicalism or liberalism, to demand redress for past wrongs. Such an enterprise by its nature demands an historical perspective. Yet such a perspective risks reifying the *opinions* of individual historians as 'fact', as a glance at competing accounts of the squabbles about lesbians in the US Women's Liberation Movement in the 1960s and 1970s suggests.

But perhaps most important is the fact which we have already noted; the fact that an historical approach renders untenable the essentialist model of homosexuality. It quickly becomes clear that 'lesbian' is not a chronologically transferable term, that it is, in the literal meaning of the word, anachronistic. Lesbian identity is a recent historical phenomenon. The notion of individual fulfilment is itself a recent phenomenon, and for an individual to be able even to think in terms of sexual pleasure and emotional intimacy very many social, cultural and material circumstances must combine (Giddens 1992). Thus d'Emilio suggests that '[d]uring the second half of the nineteenth century, the momentous shift to industrial capitalism provided the conditions for a homosexual and lesbian identity to emerge' (d'Emilio 1983). For women, of course, their material dependency on men was reinforced by the development of industrial capitalism and the subsequent segregation of gender roles which accompanied the division between waged labour and domestic labour. Lesbian relationships were all but impossible until relatively recent social and political changes enabled some women to live independently of men (Faderman 1991). Global patterns of inequality continue to restrict the sexual/emotional choices open to women around the world. All of these factors amount to a less than stable ontological foundation for personal survival and political struggle! It takes a certain kind of confidence *consciously* to embody an anachronistic identity (it is, of course, in the nature of things that everyone does just that *unconsciously* all the time), especially when that identity is under attack here and now.

What historicism offers lesbians is an account of a past fragility which does little to ameliorate the fragility of contemporary lesbian existence. With our identity fragmented by the chic postmodernity of Queer, scorned by the dominant heterosexual majority, contested and manipulated by feminists and demonised by most of the world's major religions, it is of little comfort to be told that we didn't exist in any meaningful way before the sexologists invented us! Hardly surprising then that a strand of lesbian history-telling has developed which constructs as mythical and glorious a past for dykes as any Victorian history book constructed for the Sons of Empire.

Paradigmatic of this nourishing genre is Judy Grahn, US lesbian poet whose *Another Mother Tongue: Gay Words, Gay Worlds* (1984) delves into myth and legend to uncover the etymological mythography of words like 'dyke', 'faggot' and 'gay' and weave a romantic lesbian and gay history stretching from classical Greek times through Boadicea and Penthisilea to pre-colonial Native American tribal lore. This is the stuff of myth, not 'hard fact', but it is certainly no more mythical than much that is taught in schools as historical fact.

CONCLUSION

Lesbian history is necessary on many levels to lesbians and to lesbian studies. It enables the rewriting of individual lesbian stories against their continual erasure from the historical record. It constructs a plurality of lived lesbianisms and, hence, enriches lesbian possibility when set against the narrow and demonised discursive structurations of lesbianism deployed by and in the interests of, the heteropatriarchy. It supports and reinforces the deconstruction of lesbian identity without denying the achievements of individual women who have lived well as lesbians. It identifies the mechanisms whereby lesbian existence has been suppressed, exposing that suppression (and, with it, the entire narrative process of history) as contingent and partial. It enables lesbians to construct, self-consciously, an oppositional set of historical narratives and to establish archival strategies to resist the continued denial and obliteration of lesbian existence. It is an essential tool for lesbian survival, and an essential ingredient in the theoretical development of lesbian studies. Indeed, I would like to make use of it myself in the next chapter, to give an overview of some of the key theoretical models of sexuality.

NOTES

1 Of course, I am not suggesting here that covert anti-lesbian feeling is altogether absent from apparently more neutral accounts of Sappho. Presumably, each writer who approaches her has some investment in either proving or disproving her lesbianism.
2 A lesbian relationship being seen by these writers as 'impure' by implication?

Chapter 4

What is this thing called?
Models of sexual identity

The very idea of a *sexual* identity is an ambiguous one. For many in the modern world – especially the sexually marginal – it is an absolutely fundamental concept, offering a sense of personal unity, social location, and even at times a political commitment.

(Weeks 1987: 31)

We are clearly a multi-sexed species which has its sexuality spread along a vast fluid continuum where the elements called male and female are not discrete.

(Andrea Dworkin 1988: 183)

If history shows lesbian identity to be a contingent fiction, the history of the development of that fiction reveals the operations of power through discourse in a peculiarly translucent way, as Foucault and others have recognised. Indeed, the struggles over the notion of sexual identity threaten to destabilise not only disciplinary boundaries but also the foundational premises of science itself and the cognitive frameworks on which (certainly modernist) concepts of identity are constructed. A can of worms indeed.

In this chapter I want not only to outline a queer feminist critique of the content and history of proliferating models of sexual identity (specifically homosexual identity), but also to interrogate both the theories themselves *and* the ideological and sociological positioning of the larger intellectual enterprises which each represents. My aim is not to adjudicate between theories of sexual identity but to question the usefulness of the concept itself and to identify the social and political matrices within which and by which lesbian sexual identity 'makes sense'. As the front cover of a recent issue of *Discourse* suggests, the questions which 'make sense' in the context of lesbian studies are not those concerning the causes or nature of homosexuality as a human condition – 'Is this child gay?' – but those which concern the causes and nature of homosexuality as a construct, an organisational category – questions such as 'How do we know?' 'Why do we want to know?' 'Who makes up these questions?' 'Where do these questions get asked?' 'Who gets to ask them?' (Kader and Piontek 1992).[1] What I am concerned with here is why lesbian desire is a problem which requires the construction of theoretical models of 'sexual identity', and how such models are informed by and reinforce different sets of 'truth claims' about the self 'in' the world.

BETWEEN THE DEVIL AND THE ANALYST'S COUCH

In the Middle Ages if people were not happy with the sexual behaviour of one of their number, he or she was likely to be tortured and burned at the stake in an attempt to destroy the demons which threatened not only the individual concerned but his or her whole community (Daly 1979). Indeed, male sexual anxiety appears to have been the major motivating force behind the mass slaughter of women during the witch burnings; the *Malleus Maleficarum* or 'Hammer of Wrongdoing' (Kramer and Sprenger 1486), a sort of witchfinder's handbook, is preoccupied with male impotence, the real or imaginary loss of the penis and the temptations of incubi and succubi.

The medical profession has today replaced the clergy in attempting to solve a problem which clearly still seems to threaten not only the individual but the whole community. Feminists of the nineteenth century identified 'the elevation of the medical profession into a new priestly caste' (Weeks 1985: 78), and it is now a widely accepted understanding among social historians as well as (and including) feminists that the institutional locus of social control in Western culture underwent a relatively recent shift from the church to medicine (Daly 1979, Foucault 1976, Oakley 1976, Weeks 1985). This historical process has its continuing legacy in the moralistic subtext of medical practice, what Frank Mort (1987) calls 'medico-moral politics', and as such has particular implications for sexuality. The discursive displacement of sexuality from the ecclesiastical to the medical paradigm – from notions of sin to notions of sickness – was a prerequisite for the development of the modern idea of 'sexual identity'. It also underlay dramatic changes in the public perception of deviant sexual behaviour, the treatment of those who indulged in such behaviour, and the self-perception of such people.

It is hard to overstate the significance of this relocation of control and the importance of the fact that, in common with all such displacements, its effects are far from absolute but are, rather, a function of continuing struggle. Although medicine is currently the privileged discourse within and by which notions of what is or is not 'normal' human behaviour are legislated, its legitimacy is increasingly challenged by those who recognise and contest the ideological subtext of its discourse and practices. This challenge, unsurprisingly, is mounted from within precisely those social groups constructed and controlled by and within the medical paradigm: the disabled, women, people of colour, the 'mentally ill', lesbians and gay men. The intersections among the medical constructions of these groups – such that women are seen to be mentally unstable, people of colour to be sexually deviant, lesbians and gay men to be mentally ill, disabled people to be asexual, etc. – demonstrate in and of themselves the processes of social control which are implicit in the medical project.

Neither is it the case that the religious paradigm has been universally replaced by the medical. Indeed, there has been a resurgence of doctrinally based religious activism in the United States and Europe as well as in the anti-imperialist Islamic states of the Middle East, and such fundamentalism maintains its adherence to the religious paradigm, whereby unacceptable sexual behaviour is constructed as sinful. Such fundamentalism, moreover, willingly takes it upon itself to police the practice of medicine, as the campaigns of attrition against abortion clinics in the USA and elsewhere attest. Nor is it appropriate to understand medicine and religion as being in polar opposition. Rather, religious belief continues to inform and guide many medical practitioners (the first hospitals were, after all, religious establishments), while the religious fundamentalists of the New Right make use of quasi-medical models of sexuality (Weeks 1985) when it suits their purpose. This mutuality has been present throughout the centuries' long history of the struggle between scientific rationality and religious faith, despite the tendency for scientists since Hypatia of Alexandria to lose their lives to religious fanaticism. Interestingly, the authors of the *Malleus Maleficarum* frequently compare their work to that of surgeons, claiming that it is of the same character but somehow more difficult, as this advice on the torture of suspects shows:

> The Judge should act as follows in the continuation of the torture. First he should bear in mind that, just as the same medicine is not applicable to all the members, but there are various and distinct salves for each several member, so not all heretics . . . are to be subjected to the same method of questioning, examination and torture. . . . Now a

surgeon cuts off rotten limbs and mangy sheep are isolated from the healthy; but a prudent judge will not consider it safe to bind himself down to one invariable rule in his method of dealing with a prisoner who is endowed with a witch's power of taciturnity . . .

(Kramer and Sprenger 1486: 473)

Thus, while it remains true that in the West we look to scientific medicine to tell us the 'truth' about sexuality, and are more likely to consult a doctor than a priest or rabbi when we experience sexual problems, the two contradictory paradigms must be understood as existing in continued mutual interpenetration. This is not to deny the hegemony of science and, in particular, of Western scientific medicine (Doyal with Pennell 1979), but rather to understand it as mapped on to and partaking of the ages old cultural and moral imperatives of the Judaeo–Christian tradition.

SEXUAL MODELS: SEXUAL MUDDLES

Homosexuality presents a problem for Western scientific thought. A religious understanding of the world is happy with (indeed, in need of) mysteries: the opacity of divine will, the unfathomable motivations of demons, temptation and sin. If the ways of God were comprehensible, God would not be God. Post-enlightenment science assumes mystery and opacity to be temporary or contingent – either a challenge to be overcome by the progress of human knowledge or a function of viewpoint.

Control of (homo)sexuality is implicit in the rationalist project of modernism. Because homosexuality is seen as a threat to social organis-ation, there is also a deeply felt need to understand what a homosexual *is* and how to recognise one. How to distinguish between 'real' and 'situational' or 'compensatory' homosexuality is a question which informs, for example, much psychoanalytic theory (for example, Isay 1989: 94–109). The modernist project of understanding has lead to a multiplicity of models of sexual identity, the most influential of which I shall briefly examine here.[2] There is, unsurprisingly, a glaring gender deficiency in all models of sexual identity, none of which have ever managed to do more than tack lesbian sexuality on to a more or less inadequate model of male homosexuality. Exposure of this deficiency is central to a feminist lesbian critique of current models of sexual identity. I am forced, however, to approach these models on their own andro-centric and phallocentric terms and to discuss them for what they are – attempts to explain *homosexuality*.

IT'S ALL IN THE MIND

Undoubtedly the most influential recent model of sexual identity has been the psychoanalytic one of Freud and his followers. The radical proposition of psychoanalysis was that sexual identity, rather than being 'natural' or inherent in human instinct or biochemistry, is acquired or achieved as a result of childhood experiences and fantasies within the (heterosexual nuclear) family. Adult sexual feelings may be traced back to an original moment in the drama of childhood – a childhood constructed as a kind of smithy wherein the personality with its anxieties, neuroses, perversions and psychoses is forged.

While psychoanalysis was undoubtedly a radical and potentially liberatory intervention (see Weeks 1985 for an assessment of the radical impact of Freud's work), it later became (and, despite dissensus within the profession, continues to be) a powerful tool in the hands of those who seek to discredit and suppress queer desires and behaviours. Indeed, it has proved to be the most effective means of controlling behaviour and quelling political dissent since the Spanish Inquisition and has been increasingly recognised as such (Masson 1990, Newman 1992, Szasz 1974, Ussher 1991). Masson, for example, refers to psychiatry (which had until recently a purely medical model of mental illness) as 'intrusive, destructive and vicious' (Masson 1990: 39). Psychiatric practices such as the use of psychotropic drugs and electro-convulsive therapy have been regarded with growing suspicion since the growth of the anti-psychiatry movement in the early 1960s, and the survivors of psychiatric institutions have spoken out with growing confidence against the abuses which they have suffered (Brandon 1981).

Psychoanalysis, while appearing to offer a more humane response to distress than the biochemical solutions of classic psychiatry, is thought by many to be equally complicit in the project of social control – a project necessarily political in scope. Feminists have identified psychology and psychiatry as important both ideologically and practically in the oppression of women (Daly 1979, Showalter 1985, Ussher 1991), while lesbian feminist writers Celia Kitzinger and Rachel Perkins (1993) suggest that the psychoanalytic paradigm is particularly harmful to lesbians and to lesbian feminism. Yet Freud's theories about sex and sexuality have been so thoroughly absorbed into Western thought that it is now almost impossible to imagine sexuality outwith the Freudian model of unconscious drives, repressions and neuroses (Wood 1993), while phrases such as 'Oedipus complex' or 'penis envy' have passed into everyday language. Indeed, one influential strand within feminism is devoted to feminist re-readings and reworkings of Freudian theory. What, then, does the psychoanalytic model tell us about lesbians?

There is little in Freud's work about lesbians, although at least one commentator identifies his work on lesbianism as seeming 'to catalyze his work on theories of general sexuality' (Roof 1991: 176). It is commonly agreed that in what is probably his best-known case, that of 'Dora', Freud's masculine ego/insecurity caused him to fail to recognise that her lesbian desire for the wife of 'Herr K' was a more significant motivating factor than her supposed desire for her father (Roof 1991: 175). Freud himself reached this conclusion after 'Dora' had terminated her analysis in frustration at his constant and wilful misinterpretation of her words. He also described in 1920, twenty years later, in *Psychogenesis of a Case of Homosexuality in a Woman* (in Roof 1991) his unsuccessful psychoanalysis of a lesbian. Freud viewed homosexuality with ambivalence. He did not consider it an illness and thought all human beings basically bisexual, regarding heterosexuality as being an equally problematic limitation of object-choice and as much in need of explanation as homosexuality;

> From the point of view of psycho-analysis the exclusive sexual interest felt by men for women is also a problem that needs elucidating and is not a self-evident fact based upon an attraction that is ultimately of a chemical nature.
>
> (Freud, 1905)

This equal problematising of hetero- and homosexuality has the potential to disrupt the stubborn binaries of sexual categorisation in Western thought but was sadly defused by Freud's uncompromising adherence to the binary of gender and to the unquestioned narrative of heterosex. Thus, at what Freudians term the 'Oedipal stage', young girls supposedly transfer their desire from their mother to their father and replace their own lost penis with the desire for a baby (preferably male), while young boys replace desire for the mother and wish to murder and usurp the father with desire for other women and a wish to become *like* the father. There is no suggestion that this complex mythology is anything other than a 'natural' developmental process, while homosexuality, it is suggested, results from a malfunction of or interference with this 'natural' sequence of events. Thus, although homosexuality and heterosexuality are both seen as being in need of explanation, one is achieved by a process unquestioningly 'normal', the other by an abnormality in that process. Just *why* young girls should feel desire for their fathers or young boys for their mothers is never problematised. Heterosexuality remains the unquestioned definitional norm, and the radical potential of Freud's theorising runs aground on his inability to critique the gender relations of his culture and his time. Moreover, Freud's is a gender binary remorselessly structured around the primacy of the penis, a heteropatriarchal phallacy which renders *female* sexual subjectivity and agency peculiarly inconceivable.

For Freud, the development of sexual identity is fundamentally shaped for both sexes by the idea of castration. Every little boy, he claims, is subject to, and must resolve, his fear of being castrated, while every little girl, recognising herself as already castrated, is subject to and must resolve her envy of those who are in ownership of a penis. '[H]er whole development may be said to take place under the colours of envy for the penis' (Freud, in Weeks 1985: 140). One Freudian explanation for male homosexuality is that the fear of castration has not been resolved, so that a woman is feared both as castrated man and as potential castrator – *vagina dentata*, the cunt with teeth. Lesbianism, of course, is reduced to unresolved penis envy or an arrested Oedipal/ Electra stage.[3]

Freud has been rejected outright by those on every point of the political spectrum. Right wing writer Roger Scruton (1986) sums up Freud's work as 'speculative nonsense', while Karl Popper dismisses it as simply bad science (in Ruse 1988). And certainly it is difficult for anyone with a grasp of historical or cultural diversity to take penis envy or the Oedipus complex seriously. To do so would mean suggesting that the familial and sexual customs of nineteenth-century, middle-class Vienna are and have always been universal human behaviours. Belief in penis envy as a motivating factor in human sexual development requires one to believe that all middle-class Viennese children (even girls without brothers), and all children in all other historical and cultural circumstances (even in families with dead or absent fathers), would *see* a penis, believe it to be more significant than (say) the maternal breast and would interpret the vulva, clitoris and vagina as an absence of penis. If we are to interpret penis envy metaphorically, as an awareness and envy of male social power, then why do we not have briefcase envy, moustache envy or collar-and-tie envy?[4] All of these were surely more visible attributes of male power in nineteenth-century Vienna than the penis of the *pater familias*? Only a culture (or an individual) truly obsessed with (or frightened about) the penis could construct as unlikely a theory as penis envy, and I would suggest that its somewhat startling respectability reflects interestingly on the concerns and insecurities of the middle-class, white, male elite which legitimates theory in the West.

Despite the overt ethnocentrism of his theories, and despite mounting evidence that Freud himself manipulated and misrepresented details of his cases to fit his theories and that his 'treatment' of clients was often what would now be thought of as abusive and destructive (Wood 1993), theories of sexuality rooted in Freudian psychology remain extremely powerful. It is easy to see why this might be, given the positioning of lesbians and gay men within and by a deeply anxious and repressive heterosexist society. The construction of sexual identity as a personal characteristic resulting from childhood experiences and hence, although not innate, fixed from a very early age and yet possibly amenable to later expert intervention, has obvious appeal for both homophile and homophobe.

Those who, for whatever reason, wish to eradicate homosexuality, simply abandon Freud's premise of universal bisexuality and concentrate on rectifying the wrong done during early development. This position, as exemplified by C. W. Socarides, an (in)famous theorist of homosexuality, requires a non-innate, manipulable sexuality:

> One of the major resistances [to psychotherapy] continues to be the patient's misconception that his disorder may be in some strange way of hereditary or biological origin or, in modern parlance, a matter of sexual 'preference' or 'orientation', that is, a normal form of sexuality. These views must be dealt with from the beginning.
> (Socarides 1979, in Weeks 1985: 150)

This passage neatly demonstrates the discursive location of therapeutic power, which lies (in both senses of the word) precisely in the therapists' claim to know a 'truth' about the therapee which is hidden from or often directly contradictory to the therapee's own always-already inauthentic self-knowledge (Masson 1990). The language of de-legitimation is deliberate – 'the patient', 'misconception', 'in some strange way', 'disorder' – and the discursive denial of the therapee's experiential reality, his lived experience and self assessment, is total. This claim to privileged knowledge of the self of the other is based on the concept of the unconscious mind and its supposedly universal workings.

It is important to remember that the exemplar of this strategy is Freud's refusal to believe the testimony of his women patients that they had suffered sexual abuse as children (Masson 1990, 1992, Wood 1993). Freud and his peers were unable to tolerate the implications for middle-class masculinity of such widespread abuse so, after much indecision, Freud chose to reverse the meaning of these women's accounts and told them that their memories of abuse were no such thing but were rather fantasies woven around their own incestuous desires (Masson 1992). Thus, the key legacy of psychoanalysis, for a socio-political critique of its development and influence, seems to be the assertion that *nobody except an analyst knows what is real and what is fantasy.* Rewriting history, erasing living memory, renaming and imposing a 'correct' framework of interpretation on experience are, of course, the hallmarks of political totalitarianism. It is not surprising that the psychiatric institutions of the USSR were sites for the suppression of political dissidence, nor that Jung collaborated with the Nazis. What is perhaps surprising is that these events have been intepreted as the *misuse* of a fundamentally benign institution, rather than as revealing the oppressive nature of the foundational premise of psychoanalysis and psychiatry.

Yet, although many lesbians (and gay men) *do* experience their sexuality as innate, there are others for whom the psychoanalytic model appears to explain feelings of difference which are remembered from childhood and which appear to be located as much in a felt deviation from their assigned *gender* role as in remembered desires and arousal (see, for example, personal accounts in Hall Carpenter Archives Lesbian Oral History Group 1989, Holmes 1988 and National Lesbian and Gay Survey 1992). It has also been strategically useful for the lesbian and gay political movement to agree that 'primary sexual orientation . . . and sex-role identity are formed by the age of three' (Blumenfeld and Raymond 1988: 85). This argument might best be thought of as constructing a disability model of homosexuality or, as some commentators from within a competing lesbian and gay perspective would have it, the 'we're sorry but we can't help it' model (Hamer *et al.*, 1991).

The psychoanalytic model of sexual identity is strategically useful, then, both to those who want to eradicate homosexuality and to those who would wish to construct a primarily *moral* argument in favour of lesbian and gay rights. From the perspective of lesbian studies, it is clear that the psychoanalytic model of lesbian identity is inextricably interwoven with the heteropatriarchal project. It is paradigmatically phallocentric (with the later, more intensively symbolic, Freudianism of Lacan and his followers the mere materiality of phallocentrism mutates into phallogocentrism), remorselessly dependent upon a normatively heterosexual developmental narrative and utterly ethnocentric. Lesbian sexual identity is constructed in relation to a masculinity whose (threatened) hegemony is thereby maintained. The threat to the discursive coherence of the patriarchal narrative which is implicit in lesbian desire is deflected by a frantic re(con)textualising of (mobile) desire as (static) identity. By theorising lesbianism as infantile or maladaptive, as the consequence of personal history and hence the *property* of women who *are*, in some ontological sense, lesbian (that is, women who have the property of being lesbian as sodium has the property of combustion in oxygen), the desire of women for each other becomes not a free-floating possibility but a located state of being, an identity. It becomes possible to control 'lesbians' therapeutically (for their own good), and by constructing 'lesbians' as patients, clients, infantile regressives it becomes possible to control not only those who understand themselves to *be* lesbians but also the lesbian desires of all women. Yet 'lesbian' continues to be a disruptive presence within psychology itself.

QUEERING THE DISCIPLINE

Perhaps more interesting than the (already well-theorised) role of psychology in the social control of lesbians is the problem posed to psychology as a paradigm (and, in particular, as one with claims to be scientific) by competing theories of homosexuality within the discipline. For notions of homosexuality as a disorder no longer dominate psychology. Indeed, in 1973 the American Psychiatric Association, following energetic lobbying from lesbian and gay activists, removed homosexuality from their list of mental disorders, only to replace it with homophobia, which is now itself pathologised (Kitzinger 1987). Within the constitutive logic of the paradigm, of course, if psychology says there is nothing 'wrong' with homosexuals then there must be something 'wrong' with anyone who persists in believing homosexuality to be wrong, or who persists in feeling disgust, fear or hatred of lesbians or gay men. As Celia Kitzinger says, 'the degree of dissensus and controversy within recent psychological theorizing about homosexuality is potentially sufficient to pose a severe threat to the traditional conceptualization of psychology as a science' (Kitzinger 1987: 4). Of course psychology, in common with all the social sciences (Giddens 1992, Game 1991), has never attained universal acceptance as 'real' science, in particular because its hypotheses are unfalsifiable and, hence, unverifiable (Popper 1962). They are also, by definition, empirically untestable, because they deal with human beings. It would be both problematic and unethical to set up the conditions for a 'dysfunctional' nuclear family and see if homosexual children resulted. It would also be impossible to control for extra-experimental factors. Yet, as Kitzinger points out, theorists of the scientific paradigm have been obliged to recognise that such uncertainties abound in the 'hard' sciences too. Indeed, scientific credibility must itself be understood as the product of *social* processes involving power struggles, dissent, the deployment of rhetorical devices, contests over legitimacy and authenticity, and as being profoundly shaped by socio-political structures such as gender and class (Game 1991, Kitzinger 1987). Kitzinger identifies the profound dissensus concerning homosexuality as both marker and instigator of a significant challenge to science itself:

> Dissent and controversy of this fundamental nature may come to be subsequently viewed as . . . constituting a major epoch in the development of science, but it also poses a potentially severe threat to the traditional conceptualization of science itself by exposing the uncertain nature of knowledge claims and their reliance on a bedrock of a priori assumptions.
>
> (Kitzinger 1987: 5)

This seems to suggest that the presence of competing and contradictory models of (homo)sexuality calls into question the scientific paradigm itself. To explore this intriguing idea further, I now want to turn a lesbian gaze on the various biomedical theories.

DESIRE MADE FLESH – THE LESBIAN BODY UNDER THE MEDICAL GAZE

Biomedical and socio-biological accounts, like their social scientific counterparts, have been limited by unquestioned allegiance to a heterosexual norm and by an intellectually stifling androcentrism. Within the medical paradigm, as Silverstein remarks, 'homosexuality has meant inadequately masculine men and hypermasculine women' (Silverstein 1991: 107). Queer desires, whether of woman for woman or man for man, are understood as crises in *masculinity*, and anxiety about masculinity forms the subtext to accounts of hormone imbalance, chromosomal abnormality or hereditary 'taint'. Gender, rather than desire, is at stake; or rather, desire as marker and property of gender. The strange inability of heterosexual scientists to disentangle gender, biological sex and sexual object-choice has led to heterosexuality being understood as *gender-conformative* behaviour and homosexuality as gender-deviant behaviour (Butler 1993).

Thus, within this rather naïve paradigm, masculine *means* 'wishing to engage in genital penetration of a female' and feminine *means* 'wishing to be penetrated by a penis'. Sexual desire is reduced to a desire for contact with a set of genitals with a specific physiological form. It is at once alarming and comical to witness the obsessive focus on the genitals as the presumed foundation of human desire and sexual identity that pervades biomedical accounts of sexuality (see, for example, accounts discussed in Barale 1991 and Ruse 1988).

Biomedical accounts of homosexuality fall into three basic strands, all of which follow logically from a biological determinism which posits biochemical processes of one sort or another as the cause of women wanting other women for their sexual partners. The first focuses on endocrinology – that is, on the influence of hormones on the body, either pre- or postnatally. The second focuses on brain structure. The third concerns itself with heredity, seeing sexual identity as being 'passed on' genetically, like eye colour. These explanations are both supplemented and challenged by socio-biology, which prefers an evolutionary explanation based on the survival needs of the 'selfish gene'. To fully discuss the intricacies of these various theories and weigh the evidence for and against each would require a substantial book, and such books are already in print (for example, Ruse 1988).

The important debate here is one which problematises the principle of biological determinism as an explanation for sexual desire and which identifies its positioning relative to social and political institutions and imperatives. Whose interests are served by biomedical models of lesbianism? The answer to this lies not only in the theories themselves also but in the historical and political context in which they are embedded.

Sexuality has long troubled scientists. Writing *Sexual Inversion* as recently as 1928, John Addington Symonds is clearly torn between fascination for his subject and awareness of the need for moral outrage. His fascination is expressed in peculiarly apt metaphorical flights:

> It [homosexuality] throbs in our huge cities. The pulse of it can be felt in London, Paris, Berlin, Vienna, no less than in Constantinople, Naples, Teheran, and Moscow. . . . It once sat, clothed in Imperial purple, on the throne of the Roman Caesars, crowned with the tiara on the chair of St. Peter. . . . Endowed with inextinguishable life, in spite of all that has been done to suppress it, this passion . . . penetrates society, makes itself felt in every quarter of the globe where men are brought into communion with men.
>
> (Symonds 1928/84: 6)

This passage resonates with a multitude of intersecting anxieties. There is the paranoia of the colonialist oppressor, faced with a disobedient and irrepressible behaviour impossible to dismiss as located *outside* the sphere of the civilising white world. There is the anxiety of recognising what were popularly supposed to be the germs of destruction-by-decadence present in the glorious Roman Empire, on which later imperial powers (Symonds was a Victorian Englishman) self-consciously modelled themselves. And there is the spiritual anxiety of acknowledging that God's will has been made manifest in the one-time homosexual body of the Pope. Finally, there is a rather endearingly transparent phallic anxiety/envy for this 'thing', spectacularly encoded as male, which 'throbs' in cities, 'penetrates' society and is, unlike the swiftly detumescent fleshly penis, 'endowed with inextinguishable life'! Symonds reins, in what is beginning to sound suspiciously like an panegyric, by reminding his reader of the profoundly contaminating nature of his as yet nameless topic: 'I can hardly find a name which will not seem to soil this paper.'

The conflict between fascination and moral outrage, informs most modern scientific accounts of homosexuality. The imperative is clearly to demonstrate a 'real' difference between lesbian and gay bodies and heterosexual bodies in order to define and police a reassuringly somatic boundary between the 'normal' and the 'abnormal'. Early medical attempts to define homosexuality concentrated on identifying the 'stigmata of degeneration' (Haeberle 1981), believed (hoped) to be due to and symptomatic of 'hereditary taint' (Symonds 1928/84). In support of his argument for the hereditary nature of 'sexual inversion', Symonds cites the French medical writer Paul Moreau, who describes homosexuality in Ancient Roman times as 'une dépravation maladive, devenue par la force des choses héréditaire, éndémique, épidémique' (Symonds 1928/84: 119).[5]

The fervent search for the stigmata of degeneration threw up some extraordinary 'facts' over decades of investigation. Gay men were posessed of either 'an underdeveloped, tapered penis, resembling that of a dog' or an anus which was 'naturally smooth, lacking in radial folds', depending on whether they were 'active' or 'passive' (Haeberle 1981). Lesbians could be distinguised by the unusually long clitoris that 'resembles a small penis', a piece of medical mumbo-jumbo which persists, alarmingly, into the 1970s (Caprio 1954, Reuben 1970, Wolff 1973, all cited in Barale 1991). Such anxious heterosexist myth-making continues to inform medical practice today (see p. 32).

It is already abundantly clear that biomedical accounts of lesbian and gay sexuality are predicated upon a failure to comprehend sexuality as in any way distinguishable from gender. That both gay men *and* lesbians may be recognised by their posession of a special kind of *penis* exposes both the androcentrism and the heterosexism of medicine. Unable to envision sexual contact without penetration, unable to conceptualise desire for a woman as anything other than phallic, or desire for a man as anything other than the desire to be penetrated, the result is sophisticated nonsense. It also depends on casting a disappearing spell on self-identified bisexuals.

Culturally received notions of masculinity and femininity are ingrained in biology. Endocrinologists speak of 'male' and 'female' hormones (Ruse 1988, Silverstein 1991) and of lesbians and gay men as suffering from an imbalance of these. Current thinking has moved away from locating the cause of this imbalance at puberty and towards locating it in the uterine environment, where the growing foetus is 'bombarded' with a hormone mix whose recipe is critical to the sucessful masculinising or feminising of the infant and hence, by the logic of heterosexism, to its future erotic life. In fact, of course, both biological sexes have both sets of hormones, and the endocrinal function of male and female depend on both (Bleier 1991, Kaplan and Rogers 1991, Ruse 1988), so the decision to label one 'male' and the other 'female' is suspect, to say the least. It is also true that the differences between men and women, even at the supposedly unproblematic level of biology, are far from clear-cut and include a wide area of overlap between the sexes (Birke 1992). Feminist scientists have been arguing for some time that the stubborn adherence to a clearly inadequate binary model of gender is ideological rather than scientific.

The reading of queer desire as a malfunction of gender has given rise to exotic 'treatments' of homosexuality, many of which can only be described as cruel and inhumane. Between 1916 and 1921 one Dr Steinach operated on eleven gay men in Germany, performing a 'unilateral castration' and transplanting testicular tissue from a heterosexual man in hope of a 'cure'. As recently as 1961, seventy-five men 'considered sexually abnormal' were subjected to hypothalamotomy, at least two of whom were subsequently surgically castrated when the first operation proved 'unsuccessful'. Experimental brain surgery on gay men continued through the 1970s and 1980s (Silverstein 1991). Although less data is available on medical 'treatments' of lesbians, we know that clitoridectomy, hysterectomy, pre-frontal lobotomy and therapeutic rape are among the techniques which have been used (Ehrenreich and English 1979, Jeffreys 1990, Katz 1983).

AT THE FRONTIERS OF SCIENCE – THE SAME OLD STORY

The British press and media were uncharacteristically restrained when they reported in July 1993 that US researchers led by Dean Hamer claimed to have isolated a chromosomal abnormality in gay men which they were proposing as evidence for a genetic predisposition to homo-sexuality (Connor and Whitfield 1993). Research data on lesbians was not forthcoming. There are enormous methodological and epistemo-logical problems with the findings (reported in *Science* July 1993). To simplify, there appeared to be a peculiarity of the X chromosome in thirty-three out of forty pairs of gay brothers tested. This combined with the finding that 13.5 per cent of the brothers of 114 gay men surveyed were also gay, suggested to the researchers that what they had found was evidence of a genetic predisposition to homosexuality in men. Hamer and his team were careful *not* to say that they had found the *cause* of homosexuality, commenting that, 'sexuality is such a complex trait that it could not be changed or detected by looking at just one gene' (*The Daily Mirror*, 17 July 1993), but that their research shows an inherited *predisposition* to homosexuality. It would be intriguing to know more. How, for example, did the researchers control for all other predis-positions which might be linked to this finding? How do they know they have not found the genetic determining factor for, say, heightened colour and design sense, which might lead to a career in fashion, graphic art or interior design? Or for an unusually acute sense of rythm, leading to a predilection for disco music? Or for some other human charac-teristic shared by these sixty-six men that was completely unrelated to their sexuality – vegetarianism, perhaps, a subtle difference in the shape and function of the spleen, or an unusually large appendix? And what about the other fourteen men who didn't share this chromosomal pecu-liarity? Are they lying about their sexuality? If not, clearly the little extra bit on the X chromosome isn't what the researchers would like it to be.

And this is, of course, the point. In a culture where (to borrow an amusing analogy from Weinrich) petuality was as potent a social binary as sexuality is for us, we would be looking for a genetic predisposition to felophilia (cat-loving) or canophilia (dog-loving) (Weinrich 1990: 177). Science sees only what it looks for, and what it looks for is what is socially significant, because science is as socially located as youth culture or the film industry. It is only because our culture 'believes in' a polarity of sexualities that the topological peculiarities of these X chromosomes are assumed to relate to sexual desire. In other words, it is only because the whole of Western society is busy believing in fairies that the magic works. Once one dissenting voice cries out 'But I *don't* believe in fairies!' the magic is exposed for what it is, the rather shabby set-dressing of heterosexual hegemony.

Interestingly, it was the social and political implications rather than the medical or scientific which were immediately foregrounded by the press and media, gay activists, religious groups and the medical community, with immediate concern being voiced at the possibility that 'parents may demand abortions after tests' (*Sun*, 17 July 1993). Reference was made to the fact that the Nazis had posited a genetic cause for homosexuality to justify their extermination in the death camps, and anti-choice MP David Alton rushed to put down a House of Commons Early Day Motion calling for a gene charter to pre-empt the establishment of sexuality testing *in utero*. Gay activist groups insisted that establishing a genetic origin for homosexuality would advance the cause of gay rights, on the familiar grounds that if it is biologically determined then gay men are entitled to full human and civil rights.

This position, which from a lesbian-feminist perspective is hopelessly naïve, fails to take account of other 'natural' human attributes, such as being born with a physical or mental impairment, black or brown skin or with a vagina, all of which commonly mandate the abortion of foetuses and widespread denial of human or civil rights. The *Sun* (17 July 1993) quotes Richard Nicholson, editor of the *Bulletin of Medical Ethics* as saying, 'In Britain we test foetuses and abort them if they have sometimes relatively minor abnormalities', a practice which the disability rights movement has (with precious little support from the feminist or lesbian and gay movements) been contesting and identifying as genocidal for some years. It is ridiculous to suppose that identifying something as 'natural' instantly renders it acceptable, which begs the question: 'If it isn't *natural* to be a lesbian what is it?'

WHAT A PERFORMANCE! CONSTRUCTIONIST AND PERFORMATIVE THEORIES

If lesbian identity is essential, a stable component of the self with its origins in brain morphology, endocrine function, genetic make-up or developmental glitch, it would not make sense to act as if it were contagious or open to choice. Yet the legislative and social structures which aim to control homosexuality are predicated upon notions of contagion and of choice (Chinn and Franklin 1992, The Harvard Law Review 1989) *as well* as a belief in its innateness. This ontological instability is present in all but a tiny minority of accounts of homosexuality. Even those who postulated a biomedical origin for lesbianism, such as Kraft-Ebbing, simultaneously held that 'causes for it in women [include] segregation of the sexes, extreme sensuality, masturbation, fear of disease, fear of pregnancy, abhorrence of men' (in Rule 1975). This collision/collusion of competing paradigms points to an alternative reading of sexuality. As Judith Roof suspects, such a multiplicity of models suggests a particularly fearful need for meaning: 'Why should something be seen as innate, contagious, and self-generating at the same time unless that something is unusually threatening, ubiquitous or mysterious?' (Roof 1991: 240).

The internal contradictions of the essentialist model(s) of homosexuality are one pointer to a specifically *social* model. Other important indicators have developed out of comparative anthropology, feminist theory and lesbian and gay history. To be a lesbian in Mombassa or in the Balkans is to be something entirely different from the lesbian(s) it is possible to be in New York or Mousehole (Gremaux 1989, Shepherd 1989).

Social-historical research indicates that, in order for homosexual identity to develop, specific economic and demographic conditions were required. Specifically, the growth of waged labour consequent on the Industrial Revolution weakened the economic dependency of individuals on their kin, and the concomitant migration to urban centres enabled the development of an entirely new kind of individual identity. The general development of a notion of identity, combined with the gradual coalescence of lesbian and gay social milieu meant that 'some men and women began to interpret their homosexual desires as a characteristic that distinguished them from the majority' (d'Emilio and Freedman 1988: 227). Feminist historians suggested that 'the role and nature of women changes with each society' (Davin 1972, in Hannam 1993), and that the currently hegemonic model of the heterosexual family, whose ideological supremacy was predicated upon its characterisation as 'natural', was in fact a consequence of early capitalist relations of production and class ideology (Rowbotham 1973). Sexual and affectional relations, then, must be understood as primarily *social* in character, rather than purely psychological or instinctual. Same-sex desire has been institutionalised in different ways in different cultures, from the not-man/not-woman *berdache* of Native North American tribal society (Whitehead 1981) to the ritual male/male fellatio of the New Guinea Sambia (Vance 1989).

Sexuality, then, began to be conceptualised as a *social role*, akin to 'scholar' or 'hippy'. This position was outlined by British sociologist Mary McIntosh in an important paper, 'The Homosexual Role' (McIntosh 1968), in which she suggested a move from studying homosexuality as a condition to studying the social processes whereby it became conceptualised as such: 'The vantage point of comparative sociology enables us to see that the conception of homosexuality as a condition is, in itself, a possible object of study.' (ibid.: 31). 'Lesbian' becomes, within this paradigm, a social role with agreed 'scripts' and an agreed (albeit anathematised) social location.

Social constructionism takes this insight one stage further, arguing that the social making of meaning, rather than merely interpreting pre-social phenomena, is an active, constitutive process whereby 'lesbian' is *constructed* as something which comes into being by processes of description, recognition, disavowal, internalisation, externalisation and embodiment among texts, behaviours and individual subjectivities. Lesbians, accordingly, are an 'epiphenomenon of cultural interpreta-tion' (Weinrich 1990) and, I would add, of cultural interpenetrations. 'Identity', within this paradigm, is a process rather than a property. It is both located in and produced by the interface (both permeable to and saturated with meaning) between 'culture' (understood as a set of textual and discursive practices) and 'the self', understood as a reflexive process of narrativisation (Mellor and Shilling 1993).

Social construction, whether of gender or sexuality, is a far from neutral process. Rather it is always already marked with, and in a political relation to, struggles over power. The social construction of 'woman' as weak, emotional, unintelligent, etc. is integral to the reflec-tion and reproduction of male supremacy and constitutive of heterosexual hegemony. Likewise, the construction of 'lesbian' as absence or failure in relation to masculinity is integral to the continued hegemony of both masculinity and the heterosexuality by and within which male supremacy is assured (Roof 1991).

THE RETURN OF THE DECONSTRUCTED

A simplistic reading of social constructionism suggests that, by reducing lesbian and gay identities to a mere 'epiphenomenom of cultural inter-pretation', the reality of lesbian and gay experience and of lesbian and gay oppression are somehow denied, and the fight against that oppres-sion disempowered. In fact, the reverse is the case. Constructionism does not argue that lesbian and gay identities are 'only' social con-structs. Rather, as Diana Fuss explains:

> [A] constructionist view of homosexual identity opens the door to studies of the production of *all* sexual identities, including (and crucially) heterosexuality; for the constructionist, heterosexuality is not 'natural' or 'given', any more than non-hegemonic sexual classifications.

> (Fuss 1989: 108)

Indeed, in contrast to the normative heterosexist assumptions of psychology and biomedicine, a constructionist model of sexual identity makes it possible to denaturalize heterosexuality and to engage with the *functionalism* implicit in hegemonic constructs of consecrated and execrated sexualities. Put simply, if the polarity gay/straight is understood to be an artefact, we are enabled to ask whose interests it serves. The same question may be asked of gender or, indeed, of race, disability, age or any other discursive agent of oppression. Hacking (1990) suggests the phrase 'dynamic nominalism' to describe the fluid and strategic relationship of lesbians and gay men to the naming of sexual identity, and this is, I suggest, the most useful and accurate model of sexuality currently available.

Far from undermining the struggles of oppressed groups, social constructionism offers the potential for a complete disintegration of the matrices within which and by which the binary relations of superordination and subordination are established. It also, of course, offers a model of identity as multiple, fluid and active, enabling lesbian activism to develop a politics of dynamic nominalism, which is less likely to stereotype or to exclude than the old, unsatisfactory identity politics.

For example, the lesbian mothers of one study (Kirkpatrick 1987, in Green and Bozett 1991) felt that 'motherhood, not sexual orientation was the single most salient factor in [their] identity'. For lesbians of colour, too, a monolithic lesbian identity is inadequate:

> If I could take all my parts with me when I go somewhere and not have to say to one of them, 'No, you stay home tonight, you won't be welcome', because I'm going to an all-white party where I can be gay, but not Black. Or I'm going to a Black poetry reading, and half the poets are anti-homosexual, or thousands of situations where something of what I am cannot come with me.
>
> (Parker 1978: 11)

Only by engaging with such contingent multiple identities may lesbians develop a politics which draws upon the strengths of the fragmentary and diverse meanings of 'lesbian' rather than the otiose and enervating compulsion to police the one true, politically correct identity.

The implications for lesbians are profound. Dynamic nominalism enables radical re-readings of cultural practices such as butch/femme, gender fuck and drag. Once gender is seen as a *performance* rather than the natural property of people with specific sets of genitals, heterosexual supremacy is radically decentred. And who knows better than drag queens that gender is performative (Butler 1990, RuPaul 1993[6]), who knows better than a bull dagger that masculinity is up for grabs and that a dyke can have/be *both sexes at once* (Nestle 1992). And who knows better than a butch just *how* fragile is the link between masculinity and a penis: 'He was in a rage because this bull dyke was neither male nor female. I'd eclipsed his gender boundaries' (Cordova 1992).

From a social constructionist perspective, and one informed by a political awareness (whether radical feminist or queer) which is disobedient to the doctrine of heterosexual supremacy, the foundational mythology of psychological and biomedical accounts of homosexuality is exposed as heterosexist and patriarchal. Such accounts, saturated with an unquestioned phallocentricity and dependent on the intellectually moribund doctrine of heteropolarity, appear from this new paradigm of eccentricity both corrupt and naive. It will be clear from the argument of this chapter that I see feminism as both informing and benefiting from the theoretical insights and political implications of Hacking's dynamic nominalism. Yet feminism has been as divided as the lesbian and gay movement over the issue of constructionism and has, in addition, demonstrated a deeply mistrustful and ambivalent attitude to lesbians. The issues raised by this ambivalence are ones I want to explore in the next chapter.

NOTES

1 Disappointingly, these questions are not addressed by the articles in this special Lesbian and Gay Studies issue of *Discourse*.
2 For a more detailed overview of these models, the reader is recommended to Ruse (1988) *Homosexuality: A Philosophical Enquiry* or Weeks (1985) *Sexuality and its Discontents*.
3 Although at least one Freud-influenced account of lesbianism explains it as a weaning trauma, whereby the clitoris is seen as a substitute for the lost nipple of the maternal breast. This has always seemed to me to be a particularly gripping piece of folly. First, if you want a nipple women have two real ones, so what exactly prompts the traumatised nipple-seeker to go for the genitals? Second, sucking a penis would surely provide a more accurate simulacrum of suckling; not only is it relatively the right size (if you are thinking of a nipple in a baby's mouth) but also, in the end, you get funny-tasting milk out of it. Of course the male anxiety which gives rise to such frank idiocy is above all concerned to defuse the threat of lesbian sexuality by replacing mature female erotic desire with an infantile desire for food.
4 A Freudian would undoubtedly retort that briefcase, moustache or collar-and-tie envy would simply be *misplaced* or displaced penis envy. Which begs the question and misses the point. Just how visible *was* father's penis in nineteenth-century, middle-class Vienna?

5 Symonds, in the best tradition of academics rendering their juicy bits decently obscure to protect the sensibilities of the uneducated, does not translate. My own command of French is just about sufficient to allow me to hazard, 'a diseased depravity which from the strength of things, has become hereditary, endemic, epidemic'.

6 RuPaul, Black superstar drag queen said in an interview on BBC Radio 1:

> 'I'm not a female impersonator. Women don't wear clothes like this. Only drag queens wear clothes like this. There are women drag queens, I mean like Patti LaBelle or Dolly Parton or Cher. . . . It's all drag. If you were going to work on Wall Street . . . you'd wear a three piece suit. . . . I do other drag. I do my lesbian drag – that's a pair of jeans and a T shirt. That's what I wear when I'm riding to the airport.'
>
> (RuPaul 30 August, 1993)

A thumb-nail outline of the theory of performative gender/sexual identity!

Chapter 5

Orthodoxy within disobedience:
Lesbians and feminists

Never let your oppressor define you – that's what has hurt us all along
(CLIT Collective 1974)

The subject of lesbianism is
very ordinary; it's the question
of male domination that makes everybody
angry.

(Grahn 1983)

DISOBEYING 'MOTHER FEMINISM' – A HISTORY OF DIVISIONS

The relationship between lesbians and feminists has never been straightforward. It has always been marked by competing meanings of 'lesbian' and 'feminist' and the struggles for control and ownership of those meanings. One consequence has been the construction of 'feminism' by some lesbians as a coercive and oppressive dogma. It is important for lesbian studies to locate 'feminism' in this maelstrom of avowal and denial.

It is not uncommon for non-lesbian feminists to accuse lesbian feminists of *oppressing them as heterosexual women*. While refusing to name the feminist critique of compulsory heterosexuality as lesbian, they claim to be either more oppressed than lesbians because they are heterosexual, or to be oppressed by lesbians because, by being labelled heterosexual by lesbians, they lose control of naming:

> I remember the first time I was accused of being a heterosexual . . .
> My 'natural' sexual and emotional attachment to men was thoroughly
> attacked and disparaged by the Marxist lesbian feminists I had

naively joined in the name of sisterhood. I began to wish I had stayed in the closet.

(Crawford 1993)

Here, 'sisterhood' is disingenuously set up as something wished for by a heterosexual woman approaching lesbians but rendered impossible by the 'attack' of lesbians on heterosexuality. It is hard not to agree with Sheila Jeffreys (1990) when she comments that for heterosexual women to co-opt the lesbian and gay notion of the closet to describe their own *hegemonic* sexuality is 'an astonishingly insensitive choice of term comparing as it does the real oppression of lesbians with the discomfort some heterosexual women who are aware of the incongruity of their "desire" might feel within women's liberation' (Jeffreys 1990: 308).[1] Another heterosexual feminist writes: 'Feminism's response to hetero-sexuality has repeatedly been to dismiss it, to criticize it as a neutral or normalizing area, as a threat to women, as akin to capitalism and male dominance' (Kanneh 1993). This analysis is simply untrue. It is almost exclusively within lesbian feminism, not some monolithic 'feminism', that a critique of heterosexuality has been developed and sustained (for example, Douglas 1990, Radicalesbians 1970, Rich 1981a, Wittig 1992). Although non-lesbian feminists critiqued the power relations of heterosexuality in the early days of the WLM, a radical politics of heterosexuality has not yet been developed (Campbell 1980, Segal 1994, Wilkinson and Kitzinger 1993).

At the same time as they refuse the label 'heterosexual' (Wilkinson and Kitzinger 1993), some feminists argue that they are *more* oppressed than lesbians, precisely *because* heterosexuality is so bad for women, thus recruiting a (mis)reading of lesbian theory to trivialise lesbian oppression. Paradigmatic of this genre is Tania Modleski's discussion of heterosexual-vs-lesbian oppression:

There seems to me to be a crucial difference between telling, say, a white woman she should be aware of her racial privileges in relation to other oppressed groups and telling her she should be aware of her privilege as a heterosexual female. . . . The special difficulties faced by lesbians . . . are analogous to those of a prisoner who has escaped incarceration and, being 'at large', faces more extreme punitive measures than many of the more docile inmates. The hazards faced by lesbians cannot be over estimated, but we might remember the time when feminism deemed it no great 'privilege' to be a wife in patriarchy.

(Modleski 1991: 13)

The sympathetic reader will be confident that Ms Modleski is filing through the bars of her prison in order to join her lesbian sisters 'at large'! It is, irony aside, unclear how this sophisticated feminist thinker is able to position lesbians as 'escapees' from patriachy, especially as she later comments that 'lesbian sexuality cannot help but participate in patriarchal structures of domination' (ibid.: 159). It is also important to ask, especially since the charge of racism is too often opportunistically wielded (see Ardill and O'Sullivan 1987: 290), why Modleski feels able to refute her heterosexual privilege when she does not feel able to refute her racial privilege. My experience has been that most heterosexual feminists remain in wilful ignorance of both lesbian oppression and the nature of heterosexual privilege.

If heterosexual women construct feminism as anti-heterosexual, many lesbians construct it as anti-lesbian. The development of political lesbianism, which mandated 'politically correct' lesbian sexual behaviour, was felt by many 'pre-feminist' and 'post-feminist' lesbians[2] to be homophobic. Wendy Clarke writes of 'a time in which the lesbian identity I knew appeared to be in some danger of being absorbed by new, stringent requirements for a correct lesbian and feminist identity' (Clarke 1982: 30–9), while Joan Nestle believes 'We Lesbians from the fifties made a mistake in the early seventies; we allowed our lives to be trivialized and reinterpreted by feminists who did not share our culture'(Nestle 1987: 105). She adds, trenchantly, 'We must not become our own vice squad by replacing the old word *obscene* with the new phrase *corrupted by the patriarchy*' (ibid.: 118). Margaret Hunt foregrounds a kind of politics of excommunication, which she sees as inherent in revolutionary feminist attempts to police lesbian sexuality: 'revolutionary feminists repeatedly accuse them [sadomasochistic lesbians] of condoning, or worse, encouraging, crimes against women. They try to transform them into nonwomen, nonlesbians, nonfeminists and nonhuman beings' (Hunt 1990: 39).

Such statements bear witness to a (familiar) power struggle over naming. Certain groups of women have tried to take control of the process (and privilege) of naming and have set themselves up as gatekeepers of lesbian and feminist *identity*. The politicisation of the erotic signifies something radically different for feminists (who might also be lesbian) and for lesbians (who might also be feminist), but feminist rhetoric takes little account of this difference:

> The process of constructing yourself primarily from sexual and erotic experiences or desires is not the same as constructing a woman-identified

lesbian woman. . . . For me there is a difference and that has been obscured by the women's liberation movement. . . . My desires and my sexual practice are not predicated on a dislike of men and my lesbian identity is not to be equated with an anti-male stance.

(Clarke 1982: 206)

How did this mutual mistrust develop? An answer may be found in the history of the women's movement.

MAKING WOMYN'S HERSTORY

Feminism has been extremely important to lesbians. Lesbians repeatedly testify to the transformative effect of feminism on their lives, their politics, their self-esteem and their identity. Jeanne Cordova's account is fairly typical:

Feminism healed the core contradictions of my life. Feminism said I was clearly a woman, but that I could be any kind of woman I wanted to be, and that in fact I was 'an amazon', a kind of proud, free woman who refused to be defined by the rules of the patriarchy. This sounded great. Certainly more enhancing – and more workable – than my former analysis of myself as an unrequited transsexual.

(Cordova 1992: 282)

For many women who were already lesbians at the start of the second wave of the women's movement, a feminist analysis which included a deconstruction of gender roles offered a uniquely positive 'lesbian', around which the ongoing struggle against homophobia could be structured. It is difficult to imagine, from this point in a political landscape which has been profoundly altered by the feminist and the lesbian and gay liberation movements, just how extraordinary this was. 'Lesbian-feminism', Lyndall MacCowan reminds us, 'defined lesbians as the only healthy women in a sick society, and lesbianism as an act of resistance to male domination' (MacCowan 1992: 308). Drawn to the fledgling women's movement as an environment in which they would be not only accepted for themselves but also respected for what they represented, lesbians soon became the backbone of feminist organising (Abbott and Love 1972). The feminist milieu was conducive to many women choosing lesbian relationships for the first time in their lives, and that choice was supported in a way unique to the movement.

For the women's movement, however, the presence of lesbians was seen as a problem. Since the earliest days of organised feminist resistance, on the cusp of the nineteenth and twentieth centuries, accusations of lesbianism had been used to discredit the women's movement. From the start, the patriarchal reponse to feminism included demonising lesbianism, promoting heterosex as a means to the social control of women, and pathologising female sexuality *per se* (Jeffreys 1985, 1990). It became taken for granted that feminism was associated with lesbianism:

> An English writer on homosexuality, working near the turn of the century, broadly hinted at Lesbianism in his remarks on the Feminist movement: 'The women in the movement are naturally drawn from among those in whom the maternal instinct is not especially strong. . . . Some are rather mannish in temperament.' Writing about that period, Arno Karlen . . . relates that 'Several scientists and reformers admitted that there were a large number of masculine women and even Lesbians in the Movement.'
>
> (Abbott and Love 1972)

This association of lesbianism with feminism functions within hetero-patriarchal discourse both to discredit feminism and to police the behaviour of women in general, by casting legitimate political demands as expressions of sexual perversion. If the demand for equality in itself was seen as symptomatic of such perversion no woman in her right mind would entertain such notions. The association continued (and continues) throughout the twentieth century. In 1935 the influential German sexologist Magnus Hirshfeld commented that 'among English and German feminists, the percentage of Lesbians was high – somewhere under ten percent' (Hirschfeld in Abbot and Love 1972), while Frank Caprio wrote in 1957 that 'this new freedom that women are enjoying serves as a fertile soil for the seeds of sexual perversion' (Caprio, in Jeffreys 1990), adding six years later that 'women are becoming rapidly defeminised as a result of their overdesire for emancipation and . . . this "psychic masculinisation" of modern women is causing them to become frigid' (ibid.).

The liberal women's movement which began to grow in the USA in the 1960s and 1970s was embarrassed by the presence of lesbians. Often this was due to outright homophobia: 'Many women will not even say the word lesbian. . . . When Women's Liberation got under way in the mid-1960's, attitudes about Lesbians were virtually the same inside and outside the movement' (Abbott and Love 1972: 107–8). Later, as NOW grew larger and more powerful, lesbian baiting became a significant element in the anxious attempt to discredit the movement. One important moment was the attack on Kate Millet by *Time* magazine, following her public confirmation of her bisexuality.

Can the feminists think clearly? Do they know anything about biology? What about their maturity, their morality, their sexuality? Ironically, Kate Millet herself contributed to the growing scepticism about the movement by acknowledging at a recent meeting that she is bisexual. The disclosure is bound to discredit her as a spokeswoman for her cause, cast further doubt on her theories, and reinforce the views of those skeptics who routinely dismiss all liberationists as Lesbians.

(*Time* 1970: 50)

Some lesbian feminists recognised that deploying the label 'lesbian' as a threat to keep women in line was a strategy which worked only if women agreed with the negative value assigned to lesbianism and hence responded with the expected disavowal:

If they succeed in scaring us with words like 'dyke' or 'Lesbian' or 'bisexual' they'll have won. AGAIN. They'll have divided us AGAIN. . . . They can call us all Lesbians until such time as there is no stigma attached to women loving women.

(Women's Strike Coalition, in Abbott and Love 1972)

The majority of feminists lacked the sophistication and/or the confidence to develop this strategy, choosing instead to deny the lesbian presence in women's liberation organisations. 'Many Feminists and some Lesbian Feminists were telling outsiders that there were no Lesbians in the Women's Movement. Privately, they referred to Lesbians as "The Achilles Heel" of the movement' (Abbott and Love 1972: 110).

Influential heterosexual feminists mounted a campaign of marginalisation which at times amounted to a slanderous assault on lesbians. Betty Freidan, who famously referred to lesbianism as the 'lavender herring', a distraction from the real business of liberating women, spoke out publicly against the lesbian issue at NOW meetings, accused the New York Chapter of NOW of being run by lesbians, and was reported in the press as saying that lesbians were infiltrating the organisation as part of a CIA plot to discredit feminism. Susan Brownmiller refused an invitation to speak at the 1970 convention of Daughters of Bilitis (DOB), the most important lesbian organisation in the USA at the time. The reason she gave was overtly informed by homophobia, nuanced with a peculiar blend of ignorance and political righteousness:

Gay women had made passes at her, she said; they were over-concerned with sex and were generally oppressive in their maleness. Come march with us if and when you want to, she continued, but our

fight is not the same. You have bought the sex roles we are leaving
behind.

(Abbott and Love 1972: 117)

Even the much-quoted Ti-Grace Atkinson remark 'Feminism is the
theory, lesbianism is the practice' is, according to Abbot and Love (who
were present when she said it), a misreading of something Atkinson said
during a paper presented to DOB, in which she questioned whether it
was possible for lesbians and feminists to work together. Her remark,
'Feminism is a theory; but lesbianism is a practice' was intended to
demonstrate that lesbianism, being a sexual practice and hence neither
theoretical nor political, was incompatible with feminism, which was
both (Abbott and Love 1972: 117).

In response to such hostility many lesbian feminists separated from
mainstream women's liberation organisations and instigated what was
to become a far more radical critique of patriarchal sexuality. Small,
non-hierarchical lesbian groups like Radicalesbians, Gutter Dyke
Collective, Lesbian Menace, Redstockings and the CLIT Collective
coalesced, produced pamphlets, zapped events (including some run by
NOW) and generally behaved in ways which identify them as ancestral
to current Queer Nation activism. Their astute and sophisticated theories
also predate by many years the deconstructionist imperative of postmodern queer and the Foucauldian insights of academic socio-historians.
It was as long ago as 1970 that Radicalesbians wrote: 'It should first be
understood that lesbianism, like male homosexuality, is a category of
behaviour possible only in a sexist society characterized by rigid sex
roles and dominated by male supremacy' and recognised that 'woman
and person are contradictory terms' (Radicalesbians 1970: 17–18), an
understanding that remains sophisticated today.

In Britain, the split between lesbian and non-lesbian feminists was
catalysed by a paper given at a Women's Liberation Conference in 1979
by the Leeds Revolutionary Feminist Group (LRFG). The paper, 'Political Lesbianism: The Case Against Heterosexuality', was subsequently
published in the feminist newsletter *Wires* and caused so much bitter and
furious debate that Onlywomen Press published a pamphlet[3] which
included the paper itself together with a wide selection of responses to it
from both lesbian and non-lesbian women.

The Leeds paper set out an intransigent political position on sexuality.
Stating that 'serious feminists have no choice but to abandon heterosexuality', the paper introduced the definition of a political lesbian as a
'woman-identified woman who does not fuck men . . . not . . . compulsory

sexual activity with a woman' (LRFG 1981: 5). Using the language of warfare and betrayal they declared that 'heterosexual women are collaborators with the enemy' and went on to assert that the act of having sex with a man cancelled out all other aspects of a woman's feminism:

> All the good work that our heterosexual feminist sisters do for women is undermined by the counter-revolutionary activity they engage in with men. Being a heterosexual feminist is like being in the resistance[4] in Nazi-occupied Europe where in the daytime you blow up a bridge, in the evening you rush to repair it. Every woman who lives with or fucks a man helps to maintain the oppression of her sisters and hinders our struggle.
>
> (Onlywomen Press 1981: 7)

Many lesbians as well as heterosexual women found this offensive. One lesbian, commenting that 'it's . . . the first time I've seen feminists directly deny the principle that every woman's experience is real, and valid', expressed fears for the damage such prescriptiveness might do the women's movement:

> If we can no longer express our fears and doubts and needs and conflicts without being accused of rocking the right-on boat we'll be driven back into guilt and self-hatred and isolation, and feminism will collapse into clenched fists and empty slogans.
>
> (Frankie Rickford in Onlywomen Press 1981: 12)

Another lesbian criticised the political inadequacy of the LRFG analysis: 'They reduce the whole structure of male supremacy to fucking. Withdrawing sexual services from men becomes the whole strategy – how exactly this will bring them to their knees is not explained' (Sophie Laws, in Onlywomen Press 1981: 12). And more than one heterosexual commentator angrily pointed out the elitism (which some called fascism and others compared to religious fundamentalism) implicit in the LRFG position:

> So I distrust my own feelings and reactions, and so have to rely for guidance on my sisters to tell me what to do and how to think. And before long, there I am – supporting a new elite, those right-on feminists with the raised consciousness.
>
> (Penny Cloutte, in Onlywomen Press 1981: 16)

How has lesbian feminism been assigned a position of such immense symbolic power when the lesbian presence within feminism has always been a minority presence? If, as Rita Mae Brown (1988: 592) asserts, 'the women's movement not only pushed us back in the closet, they nailed the door shut', how can other feminists assert that 'inside feminism, lesbianism was constructed as privileged signifier, as magical sign' or that 'lesbian sexuality [was claimed] as feminism's own' (King 1990)? The LRFG was articulate and proselytising, but it was few in number and was not in a position to exert control of any kind over women's politics or sexual behaviour. So why was the response to this small and angry group of vulnerable women (they were, after all, lesbians) so explosive?

Caroline Ramazanoglu cites Robin Morgan's warning that 'in societies which encourage misogyny, women can project their self-contempt on to other women' (Ramazanoglu 1989: 190), and I believe that this suggestion, although overly psychologised and individualistic, contains a germ of truth. The 'gay/straight split' in feminism is a political consequence of misogyny. By this I do not mean (as Morgan and Ramazanoglu do) that women are nasty to each other because we are projecting internalised misogyny onto other women, but that the 'problem' of lesbianism for feminism is, in fact, the problem of misogyny for and in *heterosexuality*. It is excruciatingly difficult for women who desire men to know what to do with their recognition of men's misogyny, especially male sexual violence, and with their recognition of the central role of sexuality (including sexual pleasure) in the subordination of women.

Lesbianism, and the lesbian critique of heterosexuality, is hated and feared because of the choice it offers. Male sexual violence lies at the heart of the radical feminist critique. It also lies, painfully and uneasily, at the heart of heterosexual desire.[5] Confronted with lesbian possibility, heterosexual feminists are obliged to recognise that one way of dealing with this conflict is to disengage from heterosexuality, a recognition which, in turn, relentlessly insists that they ask themselves why they don't do just that. Choosing to remain the sexual partners of men becomes something for which non-lesbian women (and clearly this analysis speaks as much if not more to bisexual as well as heterosexual women) must accept responsibility, rather than claiming it as a natural and unchangeable part of their biology.

As I have remarked elsewhere (Wilton 1993a), the intractable problem is that the argument put forward in the LRFG paper is logically unassailable, if only on the simple level that it is difficult for the majority of women in heterosexual relationships to enter wholeheartedly into a critique of patriarchal relations of power which implicates *their* man/ men. It may be difficult to commit much time and energy to feminist activism when there is a much-loved man around who needs your time and energy and to whose insecurities in relation to feminism you may have to respond in ways which dilute your own commitment to women.

On a more complex level, it is difficult for non-lesbian feminists to reconcile their desire for men with their critique of the nature and extent of male sexual violence: 'This painful contradiction of being required to love despite all their understanding of men's sexual violence is the rock against which heterosexual women, and particularly heterosexual feminists, keep stubbing their toes' (Jeffreys 1990: 241). The need to take responsibility for maintaining heterosexual desire while challenging male sexual violence is the key to the lesbian/straight 'split' in feminism. The contested nature of that violence is also the key to the other split – between revolutionary feminism and the self-proclaimed sex-radical lesbians – a split which has had profound implications for feminism, for lesbians and for lesbian and gay politics.

LOVING THE ENEMY? CONFRONTING SEXUAL VIOLENCE

In the innocent early days of the second wave of feminism, women's liberation appeared to sit easily with both the radical fervour and the sexual liberalism of the 1960s (Segal 1994). The advent of the contraceptive pill was hailed as emancipatory for women (Jaffe 1961) and the discoveries of Masters and Johnson concerning women's orgasmic potential and the role of the clitoris were seen by Germaine Greer among others as having the potential to liberate women as sexually active and 'randy'[6] beings. 'Cunt power' was seen as an intrinsic element in the feminist struggle (Greer 1970a, 1970b), and Greer's influential feminist book *The Female Eunuch*, which contains no mention of sexual violence, is mocking of lesbian sexuality on the grounds that, 'a clitoral orgasm with a full cunt is nicer than a clitoral orgasm with an empty one' (Greer 1970b: 307). At the time, all this celebration of cunts and clits read like an uncomplicated reclaiming of female sexual pleasure.

This innocent celebratory politic could not continue once feminist researchers such as Susan Brownmiller had revealed the extent and nature of male violence against women. Rape, sexual abuse, incest, domestic violence, sexual harassment and the sexualised injury and murder of women were shown to be widespread and common occurrences, not the rare behaviour of a pathological or criminal few. A new analysis developed which named all such male behaviours 'sexual violence' and identified their role in the subordination and control of all women. Perhaps more difficult still was the exposure of an overtly and unabashedly political strategy, whereby sexologists recommended training women into heterosexual docility in order to pre-empt any thoughts of independence or emancipation:

> The masculine character type, very widespread these days, incites the young woman to express her independence and seems to prevent her from passively giving herself to her partner. . . . Vaginismus expresses their aggressiveness and serves as a revenge for their day-to-day enslavement.
>
> (Friedman 1962, in Jeffreys 1990: 33–4)

An uncomfortable politics was brought into sex itself, traditionally regarded as sanctuary from the workaday world and perceived in the 1960s as intrinsically radical ('Make Love Not War' was a serious revolutionary strategy). Lesbians, apparently, were able to enjoy sex and intimacy without these troublesome contradictions. No wonder lesbian became 'feminism's magical sign', no wonder envy and bitterness towards lesbians joined hands with homophobia in the women's movement.

Brownmiller's analysis of rape as a form of terrorism by which all women were kept off the streets and dependent on male protection, brought a new urgency to the feminist struggle. No longer was it possible to believe that equal pay and the provision of state nurseries would end women's oppression, when so many men so clearly hated women and when so many women were the victims of such appalling sadism. Chillingly, it seemed that violence and sex were somehow mutually interwoven in male sexuality.

This new knowledge brought with it a multitude of painful contradictions. Lesbian groups such as Redstockings developed critiques which located male sexual violence within heterosexuality, while other feminists wrestled with the problematic intersections of racism and a sexism which had been newly recognised as sexualised. Supporting and demonstrating solidarity with Black Power, something which had been taken for granted in the early days of second-wave feminism in the USA, became the cause of frustrated soul-searching when it was revealed that Black men were fucking white women in order to exact revenge on white men, and that white men had themselves sexualised racism by constructing the myth of the Black rapist and by castrating many victims of lynching (Davis 1982, Hall 1984, Ware 1970). Women's sexuality was being used as a tool/weapon in the conflict between white and Black *men*, and racism was somehow implicated in a struggle over male power.[7]

Recognition of the ubiquity of male sexual violence against women led to the most difficult theoretical and political problems for feminism, problems which are still awaiting resolution. Lesbian feminist theoretical responses to the violence of male sexuality developed into two identifiable strands – essentialist and deconstructionist.

A strong undercurrent of essentialism informs much early radical/ revolutionary feminist writing on male sexual violence, together with much Utopian feminist thinking about separatism and matriarchal spirituality. This tendency sees gender roles and male violence as trans-historical and transcultural; 'Our Foremothers', wrote Carol Moorefield and Kathleen Valentine, 'knew the reality of man's inability to accept women as the creators and civilizers we are. That, combined with the male penchant for violence, caused them to build their [matriarchal] societies in . . . easily defensible areas' (in Lucia-Hoagland and Penelope 1988). 'This is the year to stamp out the "Y" chromosome' urges the Gutter Dyke Collective in 1973 (ibid.), and there was much talk of 'testosterone poisoning'. As recently as 1984 Bev Jo, in an article entitled 'For women who call themselves lesbians – are you trying to get pregnant?' (note the familiar policing of identity!), claimed:

> Becoming a mother does mean: . . . that *no matter what you do*, if you have a boy, he will terrorize and attack girls and, later, adult women, and statistically will very likely be a rapist . . . that it will not be a rare event if *you* are raped, beaten or killed by your son when he gets old enough . . . that you will be playing with sperm, which is a heterosexual act (and offensive to most lesbians) . . . that the process of being pregnant and giving birth is also a heterosexual act.[8]
>
> (in Lucia-Hoagland and Penelope 1988: 317)

This essentialist construct of male violence (and of heterosexuality, which is here coded as a set of *biological* practices) polices lesbian behaviour with the twin threats of male violence and of contaminating and putting at risk their lesbian identity. It also reduces feminism to a necessarily androcidal politics, since the impossibility of changing men leaves only mass murder as an option.

This degree of biological essentialism has never been more than a minority position within feminism. Patriarchy itself was, after all, predicated upon essentialist constructs of 'natural' femininity. Black feminists argued, too, that biological essentialism had motivated the widespread eugenicist abuse of women of colour, Native Americans, the intellectually and physically impaired and working-class women, through forcible abortion and sterilisation programmes (Davis 1982). Although biological essentialism was never an important theoretical position within feminism, what did become influential was what might best be termed 'symbolic essentialism', and it was this which gave rise to the lesbian-feminist/sex-radical lesbian split.

A PRICK BY ANY OTHER NAME – THE RISE OF SYMBOLIC ESSENTIALISM

Symbolic essentialist feminism, rather than theorising sexualised violence as a malfunction in or an abuse of an intrinsically value-neutral heterosexuality, developed a critique which saw heterosexual sex *as violence against women*. The focus was, to begin with, on the act of penetration. An almost obsessive concern with penetration appears throughout *Political Lesbianism*, which contains the following statements in its first three pages:

> Only in the system of oppression that is male supremacy does the oppressor actually invade and colonise the interior of the body of the oppressed.[9]

> Penetration is an act of great symbolic significance by which the oppressor enters the body of the oppressed.

> Every act of penetration for a woman is an invasion which undermines her confidence and saps her strength. For a man it is an act of power and mastery which makes him stronger, not just over one woman, but over all women. So every woman who engages in penetration . . . reinforces the class power of men.

> If you don't do penetration, why not take a woman lover? If you strip a man of his unique ability to humiliate, you are left with a creature who is merely worse at every sort of sensual activity than a woman is.

> No act of penetration takes place in isolation. . . . As no individual women can be 'liberated' under male supremacy so no act of penetration can escape its function and symbolic power.
>
> (Onlywomen Press 1981: 5–7)

This demonisation of penetration, as well as rendering a politically radical heterosexuality always already oxymoronic, constructs a political model of *lesbian* sexuality as *sex without penetration*. Penetration is set up as the only reason to have sex with men, and as an *absent practice* within lesbian sex. This definition of lesbian sex as distinguishable from heterosex by virtue of the absence of penetration was later followed by the definition of a whole catalogue of sexual behaviours as essentially male. Behaviours such as using pornography, cruising, penetrating a partner's vagina or anus with fingers or tongue, wearing fetishised clothing, using sex toys (particularly for penetration), sex play involving parts of a woman's body seen as fetishised by men (breasts or buttocks) or sex demonstrating too great an interest in orgasm (held to be an essentially male goal in contrast to the whole-body sensuality of authentic female sexuality) were among the practices held to be 'male-identified' and hence not 'really' lesbian.[10]

The accusation of male identification was an especially bitter irony for lesbians, who had found in feminism the liberating realisation that they were neither pseudo-men nor driven by the desperate desire to *be* men. Male identification as a slur was soon replaced by a wider critique which saw not maleness but heterosexuality everywhere. Again, this was a destructive appropriation of feminist thinking. Feminists had recognised that heterosexual relationships are imbued with power, and that institutionalised heterosexuality is instrumental in maintaining patriarchal power relations. Jeffreys and other revolutionary feminists took this analysis a crucial stage further, claiming not that hetero-sexuality reinforced, constructed, depended on, or was informed by inequality, but that it *was* sexualised inequality, no more, no less. Detached from gender, 'heterosexual' now meant any sex which involved any kind of inequality between the partners. This enabled revolutionary feminists to attack lesbians by *naming them heterosexual*. 'Heterosexual desire is eroticised power difference. Heterosexual desire originates in the power relationship between men and women, but it can also be experienced in same sex relationships' (Jeffreys 1990: 299). By locating heterosexuality in any and every power differential, lesbian sexual prac-tices such as sadomasochism, bondage, or butch and femme role-play, even mixed-race or mixed-age lesbian relationships, were subject to the charge of being innately heterosexual and hence not only 'not lesbian' but instrumental in the subordination of women:

> Once the eroticising of otherness and power difference is learned, then in a same-sex relationship, where another gender is absent, otherness can be reintroduced through differences of age, race, class, the practice of sado-masochism or role playing. So it is possible to construct heterosexual desire within lesbianism and heterosexual desire is plentifully evident in the practice of gay men. The opposite of heterosexual desire is the eroticising of sameness, a sameness of power, equality and mutuality. It is homosexual desire. . . . The

demolition of heterosexual desire is a necessary step on the road to women's liberation.

(Jeffreys 1990: 301–12)

Many lesbians were unhappy with this blanket condemnation of heterosex, some insisting that 'there is something genuine that happens between heterosexuals, but gets perverted in a thousand different ways' (Hollibaugh and Moraga 1984). There were also many who were angry at what they saw as the 'desexualisation' of lesbianism, a tendency which many perceived as present in some lesbian feminist writing since the earliest days of the women's liberation movement (Snitow *et al.* 1984).

But it was the naming of lesbian sexual practices as heterosexual which stuck in the throat. Lesbian sadomasochists such as Gayle Rubin and Pat Califia, and feminist lesbians such as Joan Nestle rejected this analysis as more of what they had spent their lives fighting. Here was yet another moralistically motivated attempt to police women's sexual behaviour. As Muriel Dimen (1984) commented bitterly, 'when the radical becomes correct, it becomes conservative. The politically correct comes to resemble what it tries to change' (in Nestle 1992: 141).

There was much to support this interpretation of events, as anti-porn feminists began to launch attacks of unparalleled ferocity against other feminists. Two important crises were the attempt in 1982 to halt 'The Scholar and the Feminist' conference at Barnard College in the USA (see Vance 1984) and the fight in 1985 to exclude SM lesbians and gay men from the London Lesbian and Gay Centre (see Ardill and O'Sullivan 1987). In both cases, the accusation of being 'anti-feminist' was used in an attempt to discredit the target of attack.

Describing the attempt to stop the Barnard Conference, Carol Vance writes:

> Women identifying themselves as members of anti-pornography groups made telephone calls to metropolitan area feminists and to Barnard College denouncing the conference organisers for inviting proponents of 'anti-feminist' sexuality to participate. They criticized the conference for promoting patriarchal values antithetical to the basic tenets of feminism, and they objected to particular participants by name, reportedly portraying them as sexual deviants.
>
> (Vance 1984: 431)

Lesbians Against Sado-Masochism (LASM), the group formed in order to exclude SM practitioners from the London Lesbian and Gay Centre, added charges of racism and antisemitism to the familiar charge of anti-feminism; 'SMs often wear clothes expressing real power, pain and humiliation, e.g. Nazi style caps, dog collars, chains. This is racist, antisemitic, and offensive to all oppressed people' (LASM 1986, in Ardill and O'Sullivan 1987). In a leaflet produced later that same year, as the struggle over the SM presence in the Centre continued, LASM assured its readers that 'SM was a significant part of the "decadent" social scene in 1930s Berlin' and suggested that this deviant presence enabled the rise of Nazism: 'People acclimatized to SM brutality would have failed to notice the threat of the "real Nazis" approaching.' This is a misrepresentation of the relationship between marginal sexuality and Nazism. The Third Reich was particularly brutal in its suppression of sexual deviance and destroyed Magnus Hirschfield's institute for the study of sexuality as well as slaughtering tens of thousands of gay men and lesbians (Haeberle 1981, 1989). That lesbians, in order to call for the suppression of other lesbians, could cynically and opportunistically rewrite the history of an episode in which many lesbians lost their lives, defies belief. It also makes clear why 'feminism' is (somewhat ingenuously) assigned a position by sex radicals alongside the New Right and the Moral Majority and why it has become possible for a feminist writer to attack 'feminist fundamentalism' (Wilson 1992).

As a result of this tendency to attack 'unacceptable' sexual behaviour (and clothing) in line with a revolutionary feminist orthodoxy, feminism was labelled erotophobic and anti-sex by precisely that fluid and diso-bedient constituency which should have most to gain from feminist politics: the dykes, lipstick lesbians, femmes, drag queens, radical fairies and queers of all persuasions intent on gender-fuck.[11] The presence of SM lesbians and gays at the London Lesbian and Gay Centre was defended by the Sexual Fringe, a self-defined, mixed coalition of sex radicals. Ardill and O'Sullivan (1987) were 'disturbed by the anti-feminist tone of some statements at the first meeting of the Sexual Fringe', a tone all too familiar within the increasingly anti-feminist discourse of Queer. Gay men, in particular, who see gay male sex in a homophobic culture as intrinsically radical, and for whom the assertive and defiant expression of sexuality has developed as the backbone of the collective cultural struggle to survive AIDS, have denounced a monolithic 'feminism' as life-threatening in its erotophobia and prudery (Watney 1987).

This particular partial reading of feminism springs as much from gay men's misogyny as from the repressive tendency of revolutionary feminism and the political naivety of sexual libertarianism. Feminism is held in contempt by many who consider themselves sexual outlaws. Simon Watney is not untypical of this stance. Despite citing several feminists of contrary persuasion in support of his argument, Watney caricatures 'feminists' as wishing that 'the entire system of sexuality might be magically transformed into the likeness of some techni-colour feminist Shangri-La, all tender, feeling, oceanic, tranquil – and deathlike'[12] (Watney 1987: 74). He also describes the dangerous rise to power of, 'a monolithic moralism organised around the family unit, which remains . . . a central rallying point for many of today's feminists and neo-conservatives' (ibid.: 62). Anyone with the most cursory knowledge of 'today's feminists' would be hard put to identify one whose work demonstrates a pro-family political stance. Feminism has developed a far more radical and insightful critique of the family as an oppressive political institution than has emerged from any school of queer thought. But for all queers, 'the family' is shorthand for the homophobic moralising which inspires New Right policies. It is not difficult to recognise that the misrepresentation of feminism as 'pro-family' is intended to discredit feminism. And what self-respecting dyke wants to fade away in a feminist Shangri-La?[13]

An overt reaction to this construct of feminism as 'big mother' within the lesbian and gay milieu has been for many lesbians to identify themselves as a sexual minority and to declare common cause with gay men, transsexuals and other sex outlaws. The term 'sex radical' represents the liberal doctrine of erotic pluralism (Weeks 1986), which sees deviant or execrated sexual practices as in and of themselves politically radical acts. There has also been a recent theorisation of these acts as queerly disruptive of gender (see Adams 1993, Patton 1991). Disturbing the hegemonic status of gender by 'playing' with it is a strategy which has little time for separatism. A Queer is defined as anyone who transgresses gender rules. 'There are straight queers, bi queers, tranny queers, lez queers, fag queers' (anonymous leaflet, in Smyth 1992). The SM community in particular includes lesbians, gay men and SM heterosexuals, more concerned with carving out SM space and an SM presence in the face of universal hostility than with gender politics.[14]

The queer strategic response to gender is radically different from the revolutionary feminist approach. Pat Califia, for example, acts as sex adviser to both gay men and lesbians in her regular column in *The Advocate*, and her light touch is intended to dissipate much of the hostility which she observes between lesbians and gay men. She positively revels in her ambiguously gendered persona, commenting that, 'my own gender identity is a little confusing, even to myself' and enjoying the irony that she is assumed by many readers to be a gay man: 'My favourite [letter], which I received after writing a column defending size queens, begins, "Dear Sir, I would love to sit on all of your throbbing eight inches"' (Califia 1991: xii). This playful disregard of the supreme tool of the patriarchy is feminist heresy – or is it? Does Califia's playfulness destabilise or reassert phallocentrism? Are sex radicals and radical feminists inherent political adversaries?

DYKES WITH DICKS – THE PHALLIC FEMINIST ON THE OFFENSIVE

What does it signify for phallocentricity when a lesbian dons a strap-on dildo, or claims a butch or femme identity? Is the use of lesbian pornography in the fight against the homophobic erasure of lesbian sexuality complicit with the subordination of women? In prioritising the struggle against homophobia, are lesbians betraying the struggle against women's oppression? The answers to these questions differ depending on where you are coming from. For a revolutionary feminist, penetration *is* heterosexuality, and heterosexuality *is* eroticised inequality, so a butch packing a strap on is merely re-enacting, reinforcing, and hence an active agent in, the oppression of women. From a Queer position, she is disrupting and decentring heterosexual masculinity by claiming the phallus as her own and exposing the performative nature of gender. As such, she is embodying feminist practice (Butler 1990). She is also, according to some readings, messing with Lacan's solipsistic assertion that woman = the phallus. Is the dyke with the dick an heretical saint or simply a victim of bad faith?

At base, this is a clash between two paradigms and one which exposes the limitations of both. For the sex radicals/sexual libertarians, the principle axis of oppression is unidirectional, such that 'oppression' travels downwards from the legislators of 'good' sex to punish practitioners of 'bad' sex. The concept of 'sexual minorities', curiously indistinguishable from the sexual 'perversions' so obsessively catalogued by the nineteenth-century sexologists, constructs an ontological corres-pondence between lesbianism, male homosexuality, inter-generational sex, sadomasochism, voyeurism, coprophilia, etc. *ad infinitum*, all understood to be both victimised and 'identificated'[15] by reason of their sexual desires and practices. What this position lacks is any explanation of the origin and motive of this sexual puritanism, except to recognise its roots in religion and its expression in bio-medicine and psychology

(Mort 1987, Rubin 1984, Weeks 1985). In particular, it lacks an analysis of that vector of power which is most closely interpenetrated with the erotic – gender. Thus, although the lesbian SM group SAMOIS insisted that their exploration of lesbian SM is 'a feminist inquiry', and that feminists need to 'reexamine our politics of sex and power' (SAMOIS 1981: 8), SAMOIS has never moved towards a recognition that a politics of sex and power might usefully include an analysis of the power relations of gender. Rather, it understands gender as one of the juridical practices by which the sexual is repressed and in this is wholly typical of the sex-radical stance.

For feminists, on the other hand, gender is *the* privileged axis of oppression, and this recognition in fact supplies the theoretical inadequacies of sex radicalism. Defining and policing the discursive boundaries of masculinity and femininity are, as we have seen, imperatives clearly implicit in the cultural prohibition and punishment of deviant sexual behaviour, and many feminist (and some gay male) writers have made explicit the discursive and ideological co-dependency of sexism and homophobia (Edwards 1994, Modleski 1991, Pharr 1988). However, this gendercentric analysis is confronted (and at present rendered impotent) by the contradiction inherent in the feminist project. Once gender is deconstructed and exposed as an oppressive social fiction, what is left as a category around which to organise and mobilise dissent and disobedience? Part of the ferocity of the 'sex wars' stems from the political and ontological insecurity consequential on this dilemma.

The same dilemma faces queers, who are obliged to organise around oppressive categories whose hegemony they are contesting. The relative sophistication of Queer Theory – which I suspect springs from the fact that queers are more accustomed to problematising their identity than most – accepts the strategic necessity of organising around an identity which has been thoroughly deconstructed. This is not true for all lesbians and gay men, of course: there are plenty for whom a belief in a biologically determined homosexuality remains foundational. It is, however, a useful way out of a theoretical and political dilemma and has no parallel within non-lesbian feminism.

Both feminism and queer are limited in their political analysis and both are currently somewhat 'stuck'. The question for feminism is what to do with/about gender, specifically 'masculinity'. Strategies have been developed in response to this ontological emergency, but all have proved deeply problematic and all seem to end up by reifying the very sex/gender hierarchy against which they are struggling. Revolutionary feminism, by its attempt at 'gender cleansing' feminism, eradicating the taint of maleness, simply sets up an intense symbolic and political reaffirmation of gender. The alternative, which is to degender both activity and attribute and insist that anything done by a woman is feminine, has not found coherent expression either in theory or in practice.[16]

An alternative strategy, that of cultural feminism, has been for women to resist the ontological redundancy of 'women', to rewrite the word, decontaminated of its inclusion of 'man' as 'womyn', 'wombyn' or 'wimmin', and simply to reverse the values inherent in the patriachal regime of gender. Woman has been constructed within/by patriarchal discourse as gentle, caring, nurturing, emotional, spiritual, etc., and biological difference has been held up as evidence of her natural inferiority to man. Cultural feminism simply reverses the values assigned to these sets of characteristics, asserting that women's gentleness, spirituality, capacity to give birth, etc. are signs of her natural *superiority* to men, whose lack of these attributes has got us and the planet into the mess we are in now. For all its persuasiveness (warfare, pollution, cruelty are clearly things to be fought against), this analysis, too, ends up reinforcing the gender binary. Feminism has not yet resolved the problem of how to recuperate and/or refuse gender. Rather, where it would reject it often ends up by reifying.

So how might lesbians *live* a gender-deconstructive politics? I agree with Cindy Patton that lesbian butch/femme, along with other performative gender/sex collisions, act to disempower and dethrone masculinity: 'The marvellous revival of butch-femme erotics also reminded us that we knew how to turn masculinity on its head, and that we did not have to be afraid of these powerful transgressions' (Patton 1991: 238). Many feminists might disagree with this radical reading of butch/femme, but they would surely applaud the project of turning masculinity on its head. Patton, however, recognises the reactionary nature of a femininity constructed around fear or male identification. She adds: 'Having conquered masculinity as secret agents of lesbian desire, we must now deconstruct any female desire that insists that it must be constructed against masculinity' (ibid.: 238). So, has Queer got the answer? Is Della Grace making a feminist statement when she says that she no longer needs to photograph dildos because 'she has the phallus' (Adams 1993), when she asks for 'an audience that is not afraid to cross the boundaries of gender, identity and desire' (Grace 1993)? Was Derek Jarman an ally of feminism as well as spokesman for queers when he sprinkled his book *Queer Edward II* with queer aphorisms such as 'I wish *my* father were a lesbian' (Jarman 1991)?

Gender-fuck can only be radical if it is recognised that gender, like apartheid, is a binary around which a power differential is organised, a power differential by which men oppress women. This does not mean denying that compulsory masculinity limits all men and oppresses gay men (and lesbians). It does mean recognising the social and material realities of women's oppression by men, and there is little to indicate that Queer, dominated as it is by men, has recognised that.

The theoretical limitations of both feminism and Queer leave inadequate space for lesbians. Cindy Patton describes how lesbian pornography is 'vanished' by both feminists and gay men, both groups failing to get the point:

> Some feminist bookstores refused, with a flurry of accusatory rhetoric, to carry the new lesbian [porn] magazines. They were deemed no different than the mainstream, heterosexual porn targeted by the anti-porn movement.

> Gay men were more welcoming of this heretical newcomer to the homoerotic landscape, however, in their anxiety about the inexplicability of female sexuality, they often appropriated lesbian sex magazines to defend themselves against feminist anti-porn women and elided the important differences between lesbian sex magazines (all 'owned' by lesbians) and glossy gay male porn (with a few exceptions, owned by straight publishing houses).

> (Patton 1991: 237)

The failure of both feminist women and queer men to cope with lesbians means that lesbians need to organise separately. This is more than just a pragmatic solution to the problem of invisibility and marginalisation, because lesbians are in a unique position to move forward, in a radical and exciting way, theory and politics around gender and sexuality. For only a politics informed by both a feminist critique of gendered power relations and the sex/gender deconstructive playfulness of Queer can hope to move forward. Feminism remains stranded on the shoals of gender nominalism, unsure of how to organise around a deconstructed set of social relations. Queer remains hopelessly stuck in the familiar naïveties of sexual libertarianism, content to play at being naughty and to up the ante on trangressivity, while constantly being trumped by Madonna,[17] Vanity Fair, liberal academics and other parasites on queer coolth. Marginalised/oppressed within both camps (the camp camp and the not-so-camp camp), lesbians, as *female queers*, are the ones who are in a position to develop a truly radical politics of gender and of sex. It is no accident that the most radical work on gender and sexuality is currently being penned by lesbians.

NOTES

1 Although Jeffreys' own use of scare quotes to problematise and discredit heterosexual desire is also offensive!
2 Neither 'pre-feminist' nor 'post-feminist' are accurate terms. I use 'pre-feminist' to refer to the 1940s, 1950s and early 1960s, when lesbian organising took place in a homophile context rather than within the feminist context of the so-called second wave of the women's movement. However, to call those decades 'pre-feminist' is to ignore the clear links between lesbianism and feminism which existed during the 'first wave' of feminism, and hence to erase a history of very similar contradictions and antagonisms to those of more recent times. Similarly, I use 'post-feminist' to indicate the recent development of a lesbian movement which, although it chrono-logically follows the establishment of second wave feminism as a political movement, chooses not to align itself with the women's movement. I am most certainly *not* suggesting that feminism is dead, or that it has achieved its goals.
3 A pamphlet which unfortunately is now out of print, although Onlywomen Press are considering reprinting it at some time in the future. I am grateful to Celia Kitzinger for making her personal copy available to me.
4 Perhaps 'collaborator' is meant here . . . otherwise feminism itself must be understood as that which is being compared to the Nazi occupation of Europe.
5 I am sure many heterosexual readers will be reassuring themselves that this is a lesbian view of heterosexual desire, but it isn't. I am drawing here not only on an academic and theoretical understanding of this issue but also on my own long years as a heterosexual feminist, years in which I engaged in sexual relationships with nice men who were sympathetic to feminism and aware of the problem of male sexual violence. This is a contradiction the pain of which I have faced personally.
6 I hate the word 'randy', but after much perplexed hunting through the thesaurus on my word processor and the good, old-fashioned printed equivalent, was forced to agree (yet again) with Dorothy Hage (1972: 10) that 'there is no term for normal sexual power in women'.
7 This is not to subordinate racism to sexism, simply to suggest a mutual dependency between the two.
8 Lesbian existence depends, of course, on a heterosexual act.
9 The offensively ethnocentric nature of this assertion is exposed in an appallingly graphic way by the genocidally motivated rapes of Bosnian women by Serbs in former Yugoslavia, rapes intended to shame women into deserting their homelands and to forcibly impregnate them with Serb offspring. Although ignored by the malestream media, these atrocities have been widely reported in the feminist press see, for example, MS, July 1993 issue.
10 In case this all seems so farcical as to be unimportant we need to remember

that such proscriptiveness had a powerful influence on the sexual lives of many lesbians who were loyal to feminism, for whom sexual contact and pleasure became nearly impossible. When being lesbian is so difficult anyway, political castration and the theft of lesbian sexual pleasure is something we can do without!

11 Gender-fuck is not intrinsically radical – otherwise gender-benders such as Boy George, Prince, Annie Lennox, David Bowie, etc. would not get away with it to the extent that they do. A politically aware gender-fuck – such as that of RuPaul or (to a limited extent) Madonna – gets much closer to radicalism, but it is only by incorporating a critique of gender *as an axis of power* that playing about with gender signifiers can be more than wickedly entertaining.

12 'Deathlike'? Take that and chew on it, Freud!

13 It is also important to recognise the racism embedded in this unquestioning use of exotic Orientalism to signify effeminate sensuality, a brand of racism which some commentators see as endemic to the white, gay, male community (see Fung 1991).

14 Unsurprisingly, since consensual sadomasochistic sex is hounded from every quarter . . . although (perhaps because of its subsequent status as authentically *forbidden*) SM is currently becoming assimilated into the trash-chic posturings of the elite. By crediting SM with outlaw status it becomes PC to display a young, bare-breasted blonde woman on the front cover of *New Formations* (No. 19, Spring 1993), while maintaining their difference from the (working-class) tabloids. Because she is trussed up in expensive leather harnesses, the *NF* dolly bird is coded as a member of a subversive minority whose civil liberties are under threat, rather than as wank material for male academics. She is also scowling rather than simpering . . . refusing the male gaze? Oh yeah! None of the above in any way minimalises the real offensiveness of Operation Spanner or any other establishment terrorising of the SM community.

15 By which I mean, as I have explained elsewhere, 'brought into being as a specific type'. 'Identificated' is intended to describe the process whereby identity is constructed discursively in negotiation among the labeller and those who refuse or adopt the label as descriptive of themselves.

16 Although much of the grass roots work of feminism has been guided by this principle. Women's garages, carpentry shops, computer courses, etc. are all engaged in degendering 'skill'. It's probably time this was theorised and re-politicised.

17 And just how transgressive sexual perversity can be when it holds up a healthier section of the market economy than any other industry and when Madonna's *Sex*, a celebration of polymorphous perversity which includes a nod in the direction of all the most popular perversions, is distributed as a special offer through mainstream book clubs is a moot point!

Chapter 6

Stories and storytellers
Lesbian literary studies

> I can only enter language as a subject by speaking myself. I construct myself, make myself a lesbian subject, by giving myself a sign, which also means a signification and a value, and by addressing myself to a woman I want to [be] like me.
>
> (Meese 1992: 75)

> Wherever I am and come from, my tongue is Lesbian.
>
> (Lahire 1987: 274)

DYKES AND BOOKS

Literary studies is the most well-trodden path of lesbian studies. This chapter has proved the most difficult to write, simply because there is so much already available, so much that has been said, so much to say. Not only is lesbian literature (whatever that may be) alive and kicking but it has a healthy market. Lesbians in great numbers produce and consume books, and critical commentary is part of that consumption. This picture is reflected in the practice of lesbian studies. For example, Margaret Cruikshank's groundbreaking collection *Lesbian Studies, Present and Future* (1982) contains seven articles about lesbian literature, more than any other field of study represented in the book.

This is partly due to the generally privileged position of the written word. Western post-industrial culture, probably more than any other place and time, privileges the written word. Electronic information technology notwithstanding, it is by and through the printed page that we produce, disseminate and engage with 'culture', that evanescent phantom of collective fantasy. This hegemony is reflected and maintained within the academy, with its scholarly and hushed libraries, where consumption of the printed word takes absolute priority over the unruly and forbidden spoken word. Additionally, the gendered demarcations of 'proper' knowledge are such that literature is allowably a feminine area of study. If she must study, let her read novels and poetry rather than theories of Chaos or General Relativity. Lesbians have thus amassed a body of skills and experience in lit. crit. almost by default.

There is, of course, more to it than that, as I hope to indicate in this chapter. It is important to remember that, in a global culture where the printed word has such high status, reading is always and for everybody a political act. It is no coincidence that the world's disenfranchised and marginalised peoples are so often illiterate, nor that the majority of the world's illiterates – two thirds – are women (Seager and Olson 1986). Nor is it accidental that the WLM and gay liberationist movements unleashed a flood of writing, criticism and publishing. Control over the printed word is a crucial strategy in the struggle of any oppressed group, as both liberation movements have clearly understood. Lesbians, marginalised within both movements, have an intellectual and political need to engage with literature on our own terms.

The written word is as privileged within a lesbian milieu as it is within Western culture generally. Yet this does not of itself indicate that literary studies is free from heterosexism or homophobia, nor does it enable us to take as given the notion of lesbian literature. We are still obliged to ask the (by now catechismic) questions: what is a lesbian writer, a lesbian text (Weedon 1987, Zimmerman 1992a)? What constitutes lesbian criticism? Questions such as these, together with discussion of the implications of a lesbian perspective for current literary theory, make literary studies a profitable and exciting area of lesbian studies and ensure that lesbian studies has much to offer established literary studies. Additionally, since reading is clearly a popular pursuit among lesbian communities in the industrialised West, lesbian literary studies may be the most accessible 'way in' to the academy for many lesbians.

Lesbian literary studies has one other important advantage – namely, that it is inseparable from the success which feminism and women's studies have had in this area. Language and the written word have been from the start central to the concerns of the second wave of the women's movement and, indeed, of earlier feminist thinkers. Feminist scholars have exposed the masculinist nature of language itself (Mills 1989, Spender 1983), the role played by 'literature' in the cultural construction and maintenance of male supremacy (de Beauvoir 1953, Dworkin 1987, Millet 1970), the material circumstances of women's lives which debar them from writing (Woolf 1928, 1938), the suppression of women's writing (Russ 1983, Spender 1983) and the rightful place of women writers in the history of the written word (Spender 1983). Although such scholarship has very seldom included a lesbian perspective, many lesbian writers have been unearthed along the way. Indeed, for a lesbian reading, the issue of gender indelibly marks the issue of sexuality,[1] and, hence, although lesbian-ness is almost as suppressed within feminist discourse as elsewhere (Zimmerman 1985), feminist literary scholarship is of direct value to lesbian readings.

Additionally, there are important theoretical issues which distinguish literary studies as an area of specifically lesbian involvement. The first is that the questions 'What is a lesbian reader/critic?' and 'What constitutes lesbian literature?' sit easily with current practices in the field generally. Current literary theory foregrounds questions of readership and of the interface between the production of texts and the activity of interpreting and constructing the meaning of texts which constitutes reading, and it is precisely the interface between the 'lesbian-ness' of a text and the 'lesbian-ness' of a reader which is of most interest in lesbian literary studies – what Jay and Glasgow (1992) identify as 'the complex entanglements of identity, voice, intersubjectivity, textualities and sexualities'. Indeed, it is at the interface of the subject and the cultural/ social that the genesis of 'the lesbian' occurs. Not only that, but the whole vexed question of the intentions of the author, her self presentation *as lesbian* (or not), is paradigmatic of the question of authorial presence/absence and its relatedness to disclosure/secrecy concerning the writing self. At this moment in time, therefore, literary studies and lesbian studies are placed in a potentially rich and exciting relation to each other. This makes the lesbian literary scholar's life much easier, if only because literary studies is a set of practices less fundamentally antagonistic to lesbian intervention than, say, the social sciences, where the construction of the social subject at the interface between social policy (conceived of as a text) and the social-political subject (conceived of as 'reading' that text) is not yet a taken-for granted paradigm!

The second characteristic which makes the written text such a happy stamping ground for lesbian studies is flagged by Eve Kosofsky Sedgwick. There are, quite simply, a lot of lesbian texts around! This is to take liberties with Sedgwick's work; what she in fact argues is that the presence of gay (male) literature in the canon distinguishes the relationship of gay men to literature from that of women or people of colour. Reminding us of the familiar rhetoric of the bigot, 'Has there . . . ever yet been a Socrates of the Orient, an African–American Proust, a female Shakespeare?' (Sedgwick 1991: 51), she pithily stands such closed questioning on its head by asking: 'Has there ever been a gay Socrates?

Has there ever been a gay Shakespeare? Has there ever been a gay Proust? (ibid.: 52). To which Sedgwick's retort is: 'Does the Pope wear a dress?' The point, so pleasingly made by Sedgwick, is that 'gay'[2] men are infinitely more present in the established canon than other marginalised groups. However, of course, she has neglected to ask (I hear you saying): 'Has there ever been a lesbian Sappho? Has there ever been a lesbian Gertrude Stein? Has there ever been a lesbian Virginia Woolf?' If we are going to play with canons we should perhaps expect the occasional argument to backfire, but the point is made. There are plenty of lesbian[3] writers with a secure niche in the established canon of 'great' literature. However, they are not canonised *as* lesbian writers – in fact, their sexuality is more often than not the subject of furious dispute. Lesbian scholars must engage with the not unproblematic implications of the lesbian presence within the canon, both for lesbian studies and for literary studies generally.

This chapter will have a dual focus, on the lesbian-ness of texts and on the lesbian-ness of readers. It will, I hope, indicate fruitful areas of study in both these strands and will, in addition, suggest compelling reasons for lesbian scholarship to concern itself with literature and for literary studies to concern itself with lesbians.

THE LESBIAN-NESS OF TEXTS: CANONICAL QUESTIONS AND OTHERS

When considering where we may locate the 'lesbian-ness' of a given text we confront the immediate question which has faced any marginalised group struggling to make sense of/with its relationship to literature: what to do with 'the canon', that totemised body of work dignified by the label 'literature'. The canon is the literary equivalent of that other patriarchal totem, 'scientific objectivity', and as such stands exposed as bogus by feminist, working-class and black literary interventions, which have pointed out its androcentrism, its ethnocentrism – in short, its partiality. With the infrastructures of the academy dominated by middle-class white men, literary excellence is merely a euphemism for white, middle-class, male values.

Homosexuality, unlike class or ethnicity, appears to be no absolute bar to canonical inclusion, as the reflections of Sedgwick suggest. Nor, indeed, does a combination of being female and being homosexual. What is at issue for lesbian literary scholarship is not so much lobbying for more lesbians to be canonised, but debating the contested place of sexuality itself in relation to the canon, and the continuing *political* .

practice of the canonising tradition itself. The canon demands of the lesbian scholar three intersecting and overlapping interventions: first, interrogating the (erased) significance of sexuality in a writer's work, second, renaming already canonical writers as lesbian and already canonical texts as lesbian texts; third, disrupting the boundaries of the canonical by establishing an oppositional lesbian canon and/or rejecting the operation of canonocity entirely and structuring lesbian literary interventions around lesbian readership and lesbian community values.

Crucial to each of these, and crucially missing from both feminist literary criticism and too much lesbian and gay literary and cultural criticism,[4] are the specific nuances of the interpenetration of gender and sexuality in lesbian-ness. To partake at one time and in one body of a marginalised, stigmatised and despised gender *and* sexuality is to be positioned twice over as outsider, with all the social hazards that brings with it. Importantly, it is also to partake of the material disadvantage which accrues to women, although it is becoming apparent (Dunne 1992) that some ways of being lesbian defray certain manifestations of that disadvantage (see pp. 186–7). It has been a truism of feminism since Virginia Woolf published *A Room of One's Own* (1928) that women have neither the economic independence nor the domestic support to enable them to write. This is paralleled by Lillian Faderman's suggestion (1991) that increasing *economic* independence from men enabled women to start living as lesbians in the industrialised West. It is no accident that the lesbian voice until recently – Radclyffe Hall, Natalie Barney, Gertrude Stein, Djuna Barnes, Virginia Woolf herself – has been a privileged, or even aristocratic, white voice. The interactions of class, race and gender which make it difficult for women to write are additionally inflected for lesbians by homophobia. It is one thing for wealthy white lesbian writer Radclyffe Hall to stand up in court and defend *The Well of Loneliness* – while in no way belittling her courage and achievement we can recognise that the trial did ensure free publicity for an already published book – it is quite another for Isabel Miller to be forced to self-publish her lesbian romantic novel *Patience and Sarah* (Zimmerman 1992a) because no publisher would take it – and we have no way of knowing how many lesbians, lacking the financial resources of even Miller, have been permanently silenced. As long as the material inequality between women and men continues (and the gap between men's and women's earning power shows no signs of reducing), gay men will be better off than their heterosexual counterparts, while lesbians will be worse off. In addition, institutional racism constructs an economic sub-class of people of colour, such that lesbians of colour write under multiple disadvantage.

THE CANON AS CLOSET – REVALUING THE SPECIFICS OF DESIRE

Any reader who went to school would have been unlikely to avoid contact with homosexual literary products. E. M. Forster, Oscar Wilde, Siegfried Sassoon, Christopher Marlowe, W. H. Auden, Virginia Woolf are all staples of the English literature curriculum but their sexuality is most ruthlessly and completely expurgated. Given the quite clearly held premise that to mention the existence of homosexuality to children and young people is tantamount to encouraging active homosexual experimentation among them, this mendacity is quite logical within the context of the 'we know what's good for you better than you do' model of schooling. The traditional model of higher education, however, is supposedly predicated on the dictum that no field of inquiry should be closed to the scholarly mind, so surely we might expect an open engagement with the implications of canonical writers' homosexuality within the lofty confines of the academy? To a certain extent this is the case, but only with any consistency within lesbian/and gay studies or feminist studies/women's studies, themselves beleaguered and marginalised academic projects. Outwith these special interest areas, the expurgation is more sophisticated, but no less absolute for that. It is not the writers' homosexuality which is denied but its significance. There can be no more delightful and biting exposé of the convoluted logic whereby the meaningful is transmuted into the meaningless than Eve Kosofsky Sedgwick's. In *Epistemology of the Closet* (1991) Sedgwick lists the increasingly desperate excuses of the academic homophobe not to pay any attention to the (homo)sexuality of great writers:

1 Passionate language of same-sex attraction was extremely common during whatever period is under discussion – and therefore must have been completely meaningless. Or
2 Same-sex genital relationships may have been perfectly common during the period under discussion – but since there was no language about them *they* must have been completely meaningless. Or
3 Attitudes about homosexuality were intolerant back then, unlike now – so people probably didn't do anything. Or
4 Prohibitions against homosexuality didn't exist back then, unlike now – so if people did anything it was completely meaningless. Or

5 The word 'homosexuality' wasn't coined until 1869 – so everyone before then was heterosexual. (Of course heterosexuality has
   always existed.) Or

6 The author under discussion is rumoured to have had an attach-
   ment to someone of the other sex – so their feelings about people
   of their own sex must have been completely meaningless. Or
   (under a perhaps somewhat different rule of admissable evidence)

7 There is no actual proof of homosexuality, such as sperm taken
   from the body of another man or a nude photograph with another
   woman – so the author may be assumed to have been ardently and
   exclusively heterosexual. Or (as a last resort)

8 The author or the author's important attachments may very well
   have been homosexual – but it would be provincial to let so
   insignificant a fact make any difference at all to our understnding
   of any serious project of life, writing, or thought.

(Sedgwick 1991: 52–3)

The canon itself functions as a closet for queer authors. Of course, it
does not see fit to extend the same courtesy to its presumptively
heterosexual cannonees. Lit. crit. practice functions not to exclude *all*
distracting biographical information about its authors, nor to reject *all*
perhaps voyeuristic and salacious examination of their sexual or affectional lives. The 'Dark Lady' of Shakespeare's sonnets (rather than the
Dark Gentleman), the Elizabeth Barrett of Robert Browning, the
suspiciously incestuous feeling for their sisters of Keats or Wordsworth
are the staples of English literature. This silencing is performed on
behalf of the presumptively homosexual only. It is, then, a political
activity, and one which aligns the academy with every other institution
in dominant Western patriarchal culture in policing the arena of the
sexual. This docility marks literary studies as an incomplete and servile
academic enterprise. Is a writer's sexuality any less significant than
Sylvia Plath's depressions or Virginia Woolf's membership of the
Bloomsbury Group? Proclaiming the death of the author (and replacing
her with a collective authorial project encompassing textual production
and consumption) does not invalidate the investigation of personal
biography, rather it revalidates it. If the author is simply the fleshly
transcriber of cultural and social texts and signs, and the text itself a
temporal and contingent ephemerality in which readers construct meanings from their own semiotic codes, how much more important is an
understanding of the social and cultural contexts in which both producer

and reader are embedded! If (homo)sexuality is always already insignificant, a sign not present and not presentable, then 'text' is merely 'heterotext' and reading merely 'heteroreading', leaving those who would engage critically with texts amusing themselves safely in a sort of ideological playpen.

The intellectual price we pay for this censorship is often high. In my copy of the Penguin edition of Virgina Woolf's *Orlando* the author is described in the blurb as, 'the daughter of Sir Leslie Stephen and the wife of Leonard Woolf'. These biographical details are clearly of such significance that they are the very first words you read on opening the book. Her long and passionate love affair with Vita Sackville-West, the book's inspiration, goes unmentioned. Virginia-as-wife-and-daughter erases the significance of the novel to lesbians. Published in the same year as *The Well of Loneliness*, *Orlando* has certainly not developed the same status as lesbian classic. Lesbian reader accounts frequently complain of the problems inherent in identifying with Stephen Gordon, *The Well*'s hero (O'Rourke 1989), but reading the book has nevertheless become almost a rite of passage for baby dykes. It is intriguing to speculate what it would mean to *be* lesbian in English-speaking culture now if *Orlando* rather than *The Well* had been read as a lesbian text.

The first project of lesbian literary studies must be to revalue the significance of sexuality in the ongoing process of critical appraisal/ reappraisal of writers already accepted as worthy of the canon. As with all other academic disciplines, turning a lesbian perspective on to literary studies serves to reveal the ridiculous and intellectually damaging operations of heterosexism and enables the wider project of literary studies/literary criticism to develop towards an intellectual maturity currently denied it by the ideological/political stranglehold stunting its growth. Just as the struggles of Black intellectuals have made it absurd to continue to ignore the influence of racism on literature[5] – on Black and non-Black writers and readers alike, on the construction of a (Eurocentric) canon and set of critical and pedagogic practices, on the establishment of 'oppositional' canons and genres – so it becomes absurd to ignore the influence of heterosexism.

Lesbian questions asked of and about the already canonical must be located in our awareness of the contingent nature of lesbian-ness. What did her understanding of her experiences as Sackville-West's lover mean for Woolf's presentation of gender and sexuality in her writing? What do we get when we undertake a comparative evaluation of 'lesbian' in *Orlando* and *The Well of Loneliness* (products of similar social-political milieux)? Is it appropriate to conceptualise Woolf as lesbian, heterosexual or bisexual, given our understanding of the 'meaning' of those categories then and now? Just as important, how do we account for our private ascription of sexual identity to Woolf (and, by extension, to *every* author) as readers, and how do competing ascriptions of sexual identity inflect the process of reading? In other words, is the dyke's *Orlando* a different book from the homophobe's *Orlando*, and how is that difference significant?

SHE'S ONE OF OURS! STAKING CLAIMS IN THE CANON

Reclaiming the great lesbians of literature (or rather, renaming them lesbian) constitutes an anti-homophobic intervention. In response to those who believe that deviant sexual behaviour contaminates the wellspring of human creativity at source, or that lesbian sexuality is immature and hence not to be associated with challenging thinkers or artists, it is obviously important to be able to thumb one's nose and produce a handful of Great Literary Lesbians to confound the argument. Yet to engage on that level of combat is to enter the lists at a disadvantage. For proving a writer's lesbian-ness to the satisfaction of the cynical homophobe is not possible, given the circularity of the homophobic argument – lesbians are immature/sick, therefore they cannot produce 'great' writing, therefore anyone who *can* produce great writing is, QED, *not* a lesbian. Given the intractable illogic of the strategies of denial outlined by Sedgwick above, unless we discover a previously unknown photograph of, say, Woolf and Sackville-West in flagrante delicto with clearly visible strap-on and supporting documentation (such as, perhaps, the receipt from a well-known Bloomsbury sex aids shop?), the absolute certainty of homophobic denial is unlikely to be dented.[6] So the simple naming-as-lesbian of the likes of Virginia Woolf is useful primarily in order to enable the survival and self-worth of living lesbians. Given that the body of hegemonic cultural production constructs the lesbian as inevitably doomed, the importance of a few precious successful/creative/happy lesbian foremothers should not be underestimated, but the interventions of lesbian scholarship into the canon should take the subversion further. It is by questioning the significance of sexual identity to the processes of writing, reading and literary scholarship that a lesbian disruption of the oppressive and intellectually redundant paradigm of canonicity may be set in motion.

Your canon or mine? An oppositional scholarship

In addition to confronting the established canon with its own inadequacies and proclaiming the lesbian-ness of already canonical texts,
there is a third important lesbian literary studies strategy: the setting up
of an alternative/oppositional canon. Establishing an oppositional canon
of women writers has been one of the most important achievements of
feminism. This resistance to erasure has taken a stubbornly material
form. Feminist literary historians have uncovered a growing body of
evidence which strongly suggests that a book written by a woman is
simply a more ephemeral being than a book written by a man, and that
this is largely due to the fact that publishing, reviewing, marketing and
lit. crit. are all male-dominated. So feminist publishing houses made
available a corpus of women's writing which would otherwise simply
not *be* here.

At least one strand of lesbian political/theoretical activism has been
interwoven with feminism, and feminist publishers have done much to
make lesbian writing available. In addition, alongside the feminist
publishing houses, critical texts and journals, lesbian equivalents have
mushroomed. Lesbian publishing predates feminism, of course, as does
the existence of a lesbian sub-culture (Faderman 1991). Publications
such as *The Ladder* and *Vice Versa* were produced by lesbians for
lesbians and were established before the second wave of the women's
movement made women's publishing a feminist enterprise.

The purpose of such publications – indeed, the purpose of much (if
not all) lesbian writing – is 'to be useful' (Zimmerman 1992a); that is,
to meet social rather than aesthetic criteria, to enable lesbians to read *as*
lesbians, rather than reading 'between the lines' or 'against the grain' of
heterotexts.

LESBIAN READING/READING LESBIAN

I want next to consider the broader relationship between literature and
'lesbian' in all its somewhat daunting complexity. In order to make
sense of this complexity it is important to start from an understanding of
where lesbians as writers, readers, critics, students or teachers of literature are situated in relation to the cultural mainstream. Lesbians are a
minority whose subordination is actively maintained by social, political,
religious and cultural institutions and practices. One important cultural
mechanism whereby such subordination is maintained and reproduced is
the labelling-as-other of the subordinate by the superordinate, a labelling

located within literature and other cultural practices as much as within the discourses of law or medicine. Feminist and anti-racist critiques have identified the construction of woman-as-other and Black-as-other within literature, the broadcast media, film and popular culture and have pointed to the instrumentality of such cultural practices in the construction of Black or female (or, of course, Black female) subjectivity (see for example hooks 1990, Wilton 1992a). But there is an additional dynamic at work for lesbians – the dynamic of the closet, of invisibility and of passing.

Although 'race' is a social construct not a biological 'reality' (and although the skin colour of Black people may range from deepest ebony to Michael Jackson pale, overlapping the darker skin tones of many who are considered to be 'white'), on the whole it is true to say that people of colour are generally recognisable as such. Racism is, therefore, not something which the majority of Black people may deal with by passing as white. Similarly, outwith the blurred boundary inhabited by drag queens, passing women, transvestites and transsexuals, women are visible *as* women and do not on the whole deal with sexism by passing as men.[7]

For lesbians (and of course gay men) living in a culture which is homophobic to the point of hostility and physical violence, passing is a survival strategy they may have little choice about adopting. For others, the problem of 'passing' may be reversed: so absolute is the presumption of heterosexuality that a lesbian who wants *not* to be mistaken for heterosexual has a hard time presenting as unmistakably lesbian. Singer k d lang complained, 'I always thought I was out. . . . I presented myself as myself. . . . I did not do anything to cover it up; I just lived my life' (Bennetts 1993). Lesbians don't, despite anxious and contradictory research findings about body morphology, pipe-smoking tendencies or whistling ability (Ruse 1988), exhibit any physical differences from non-lesbian women. Unless a lesbian wants you to know that she is a lesbian, or unless you are initiated into the codes by which she presents her lesbian self to other lesbians, you cannot tell. And so anxious and totalitarian is the institution of heterosexual supremacy that even if she *does* want you to know, communication is uncertain. This is probably more true now, with the emergence of lesbianism-as-style among the purchasing classes, than at any time in the last fifty years; as shorn hair, masculine garb and even sadomasochistic paraphernalia become absorbed into the dress codes of the cool and trendy it is increasingly difficult to read 'real' lesbians with any degree of accuracy.

This complex and intersecting set of cultural practices, denying, co-opting, re-forming and digesting the lesbian presence in the social body, combines with the general cultural and social marginality of women to produce a phenomenon widely known as lesbian invisibility. It is lesbian invisibility which enables medical practitioners to claim that none of their patients are lesbian (Johnson *et al.* 1981, in Clarke 1988), feminist writers to 'forget' that lesbians exist (for example, Miles 1991) and literary critics to claim that writers from Sappho to H.D. are 'really' heterosexual. As critic Bonnie Zimmerman puts it, 'the lesbian must overcome this invisibility, a metaphysical dilemma unique to homosexuals. The dominant culture suppresses her existence so thoroughly that she may not even know she exists' (Zimmerman 1992a: 39). I want here to engage with the effects of lesbian invisibility on individual women, both as writers and readers, and on lesbian literature.

Growing up lesbian[8] is for the most part a painful and difficult experience. Young heterosexual women's sexual relationships with men are reflected, encouraged and naturalised by the dominant culture (albeit in a repressive and controlling way). Indeed, all modes of cultural life in the (over)developed West are saturated with and shaped by the heterosexual imperative. Turn on a television or radio, browse through a newsagent's magazine rack or the shelves of a bookshop, rent a video, visit a cinema, art gallery or museum, go to a concert – rock, folk, blues, jazz, classical, opera – or an academic conference, and heterosexuality in all its hegemonic lustre confronts you.[9] For the baby dyke, whether she be 14 years old and emerging from childhood or 40 and emerging from marriage, what confronts her is her own invisibility. She is also undoubtedly aware that to be a lesbian is dangerous, so this is something she must hide. This combination of invisibility and danger means that lesbian books often provide not only the first non-homophobic context within which a lesbian reader may begin to understand her existence but also the first lesbian 'community'.

Additionally, the process of 'reading lesbian' constructs the lesbian reader *as* lesbian. It is a commonplace of lesbian autobiography that books – often pulp fiction aimed at a heterosexual readership and presenting a lurid and oppressive stereotype of 'lesbian' – enabled the writer to read/write *herself as lesbian* (Hennegan 1988, Lynch 1992, Meese 1992, Zimmeran 1992a). Having a language with which to make sense of one's experience is, in an almost Lacanian sense, essential to subjectivity. As Elizabeth Meese so powerfully puts it, 'language is not "outside" me, except in the way that skin is "outside" the body. No skin, no body' (Meese 1992: 81).

Lesbian writing, then, is crucially important to lesbian readers in a way which is difficult for non-lesbians to understand. One consequence of this, and something which helps shape a lesbian response to literature and a lesbian approach to literary studies, is that the canonical boundary takes second place to the homo/heterosexual (or, more exactly, the lesbian/heterosexist) boundary. As Bonnie Zimmerman suggests, popular or 'pulp' fiction has a significance to lesbian reading that it does not have for mainstream reading, especially in particularly hostile cultural contexts: 'pulp paperbacks were crucial to the lesbian culture of the 1950s because they offered proof of lesbian existence' (Zimmerman 1992a: 9). Indeed, many of these early lesbian pulp novels are currently being republished. Zimmerman proposes a radical approach to lesbian literature which maps out lesbian fiction as a genre *per se*, rather than understanding lesbian writing as consisting of lesbian content within many genres – the detective novel, romantic fiction, gothic, etc.

> The significance of lesbian fiction lies not so much in the individual text abstracted from its political and social context, but in the genre taken *as a whole*, in its interplay of ideas, symbols, images and myths. The purpose of this writing – self-aware or not – is to create lesbian identity and culture. . . . Whatever their aesthetic value, lesbian texts are 'sacred objects' that bind the community together and help express – by which I mean both reflect and create – its ideas about itself.
>
> (Zimmerman 1992a: 20–1)

Clearly, the implications of this marking of the lesbian text as 'sacred object' are multiple and complex. Two of the most significant are the burden of expectation laid on any lesbian writing and the importance of autobiography as a genre within lesbian literature.

SACRED OBJECTS

For a people isolated by social opprobrium and stigma, made 'a people' only by sexuality, that most fragile and contested of commonalities, autobiography holds a particular significance. Unlike other oppressed groups, lesbians (and gay men) are an utterly disparate collection of people. We do not necessarily have anything in common other than our sexuality. Religion, skin colour, family experience, socio-economic class, nationality, culture, language – all may divide rather than unite us. We are not born into comforting rituals, beliefs or practices which sustain our sense of community. Indeed, we are too often ejected from our communities of birth *because of* our sexuality, something particularly painful for minority lesbians and gays. And the very thing which we call upon to construct our sense of community is itself under constant challenge and question. Just as feminism is working towards its own irrelevance by seeking to deconstruct gender, so deconstructionist approaches to sexuality and queer theory constantly destabilise sexual identity. The debate between essentialism and constructionism and the gender-fuck antics of Queer threaten the very ground on which 'lesbian' stands. Mainstream culture gives us nothing to which to anchor ourselves; nor does our own. We are like spiders making webs between clouds. The high cost of living in this cultural stratosphere should not be underestimated, for culture 'limits and organises human experiences. It does so by providing a version of reality that guarantees the shared meanings necessary for social existence' (Wahlstrom and Deming in Zimmerman 1992a).

In this remarkable existential fluidity all we have to hold on to are our stories. Additionally, for many lesbian readers, lesbians in books are the only other lesbians to be found. Autobiography then, and specifically autobiography which foregrounds the author's experience of herself as lesbian, fulfils a poignantly crucial function.

The importance of lesbian autobiography is reflected in the sheer number of books available. Among the collections of accounts from around the world, from lesbians of colour, Jewish lesbians, lesbian nuns, older lesbians, etc., are many of coming-out stories. In all these autobiographical accounts the focus is on the writer's construction of and understanding of herself *as a lesbian*. In some, the exclusionary nature of 'lesbian' is revealed by the struggle to define a self as lesbian *and* Black, Jewish, disabled or working class. Most autobiographies are about something other than a simple *human* life. After all, there has to be something interesting about the person writing the autobiography for a reader to want to read it, or for the writer to feel justified in putting us to the trouble of reading it. Most are written by people who are, for one reason or another, already famous, and the personal account is structured around the journey to, and probably the reasons for, that fame. The presentation is of an already *public* self, and the reader's pleasure is usually located in the privileged drawing aside of the public persona to reveal the private, 'authentic' self, the illusion of getting to know 'personally', a public person and finding that person engagingly (or disquietingly) human. Although this remains true for most book-length lesbian autobiographies – written by women who are already public figures in some sense – the genre of brief autobiographical accounts collected together *as* lesbian accounts are from non-public figures, 'ordinary' people, often privileging oral accounts. It is because the writers belong to groups silenced within the mainstream that their accounts are valued, and the value is psychological and social not aesthetic. Such works present a challenge to the (spurious) aestheticism of mainstream literary criticism and become part of a process of blurring the boundaries between the aesthetic and the sociological. Textual criticism is no longer enough, the skills of traditional literary criticism fall far short of understanding the significance and value of such writing.

Traditional literary criticism has less difficulty with established writers such as Rosemary Manning or Audre Lorde, who write lesbian autobiography, although traditional critics are often unwilling or unable to get to grips with the 'lesbian' in their writing. Lorde's rich and inspirational 'biomythography' *Zami: A New Spelling of My Name* (1982), with its powerful self-consciousness as a voice speaking to people who have an urgent need to hear, is 'on the verge of canonisation within white feminist academia as the token Black lesbian voice' (Wilson 1992). As Wilson warns, this does not mean that white feminist academia is confronting racism and homophobia – far from it:

> For feminist academia Lorde is particularly effective as a token: since she is Black, lesbian and a mother, her work compactly represents that generally repressed matter towards which white feminists wish to make a gesture of inclusion but since Lorde conveniently represents so much at once, she can be included without her presence threatening the overall balance of the white majority vision.
>
> (Wilson 1992: 77)

This does not detract from the importance of Lorde's work, but is a timely reminder of the dangers of ghettoisation and co-option constantly facing non/anti-mainstream writing and reading.

It is not only in declared autobiographical narrative that autobiographical material is presented. Much lesbian poetry for example is autobiographical – Audre Lorde, Adrienne Rich, Pat Parker, Cheryl Clarke and Judy Grahn all write directly autobiographical poetry – but they are doing more than simply recounting their life stories. Christian McEwan (1988) identifies a child-like quality in lesbian poetry and suggests that this grows from the power relations of heteropatriarchy:

> For years those children had kept their secrets to themselves. . . . Now at last they were beginning to speak up, to try to make their voices heard over the confident pronouncements of the grownups

(substitute *whites*, substitute *straight people, rich people, people with power, the literary establishment, the middle class*). They were trying to tell what they saw as the truth, and the grownups were refusing to believe them.

(McEwan 1988: xv, emphasis in original)

McEwan understands this childishness as being a crucial stage in the collective process of lesbian survival, a struggle against odds which 'kindly straight friends find it hardest to believe in' (ibid.: xv). Rejecting the stereotypical assessment of lesbian poetry as 'wear(ing) its heart on its sleeve (or its identity on its lapel)' she judges that:

The most interesting work is being done neither out of innocence nor in self-defence, but at a point slightly beyond, where the clear-eyed child and the outraged adult start to merge. . . . Always she acts in the knowledge of her own past pain and of the harm that it has done, and always she uses that knowledge to generate a new, more responsible kind of behaviour.

(ibid.: xvi)

It has hardly been a demand of non-lesbian poetry that it 'generate a new, more responsible kind of behaviour' but this 'ethical imperative', which informs much lesbian cultural commentary, is one indication of the kinds of *non-aesthetic* standards by which lesbian behaviour, including writing behaviour, is judged by lesbian critics. In this, it is markedly different from mainstream lit. crit. Ironically, one frequent casualty of this ethical imperative is sexually explicit writing, including the autobiographical.

Sexually explicit writing is a sub-genre of lesbian writing (see Zimmerman 1992a for a detailed discussion of the genre of lesbian erotica), and much is autobiographical. If lesbians need autobiography to construct a social self, we also evidently need sexual autobiography in order to construct a sexual self, and lesbian writers have been remarkably willing to provide this. The best known of these is Joan Nestle – self-identified, working-class, Jewish, lesbian, feminist femme – whose writing confounds genre classification, inextricably mixing historical accounts of what it was like to be part of the butch–femme lesbian community in 1950s New York with glimpses of childhood and frankly erotic retellings of sexual encounters. Nestle's writing constructs a specifically *sexual* lesbian self, and has been condemned by some as pornographic and anti-feminist.

Clearly, this response is determined by the location of all lesbian readings within heteropatriarchal culture. Whether it is to be (psychologically) read as manifesting 'internalised' homophobia and loathing of the sexual self of the reader, or (sociologically) as demonstrating a political and strategic allegiance to a 'lesbian' that is *not* a sexual category at all, or (textually) as a negotiation and conflict over the boundaries of the pornographic and the positioning of lesbian sexuality within that arena, it may not be understood as external to and uncontaminated by homophobia.

For Nestle, her experience of homophobia is mapped on to her experience of antisemitism; for lesbians of colour, homophobia intersects with racism in a way which makes their explicit presentation of Black lesbian *sexuality* doubly important, an issue which has not been fully confronted by lesbian feminist positions on sexually explicit lesbian writing. Cheryl Clarke writes, 'My everyday life as a Black lesbian writer is marked by the struggle to be a (sexual) black lesbian, the struggle for the language of sexuality, and the struggle not to be the "beached whale of the sexual universe"'.[10] Clarke, Pat Parker and other lesbians of colour choose to confront racism and homophobia by specifically sexualised writing, a strategy which has been largely disrespected by white academic feminists.

THE SUICIDE OF THE AUTHOR? SOME FAMOUS LESBIAN NON-AUTOBIOGRAPHIES

Perhaps the most famous – and intransigent – taking further of the lesbian autobiography is Gertrude Stein's *The Autobiography of Alice B. Toklas* (1933). Not an autobiography at all, or, at least, an autobiography whose author/subject is curiously deflected on to the person of her lover, it purports to be written by Alice, although Stein always named herself openly as the author. The book details their life together as American expats in the exciting world of bohemian Paris and reports unambiguously Alice's feelings of love and veneration for Gertrude. So why the deflection of authorship?

Their class privilege, Gertrude's extraordinary self assurance, her later fame and the avant-garde values of their bohemian circle enabled them to be perfectly candid about their relationship. The world was expected to take them as they found them, which apparently the world was happy to do. There are, nevertheless, hidden things about the lesbian-ness of their desire in Stein's writing. Her erotic prose is so densely coded as to render its sexual content obscure to say the least. Decoders of Stein assure us that 'cow' means orgasm and 'lifting belly' refers to sex, but interpretations differ, and this oblique symbolic language is hardly an open and accessible account of lesbian sex. Stein and Toklas have been obliterated as lesbians in the discrete unaccepting acceptance of the heterosexist mainstream. Toklas is referred to as Stein's 'amanuensis' who 'joined the group' (of Stein's artistic salon) rather than as her lesbian life partner.

Not all commentators have taken it upon themselves to erase the scandalous sexuality of Stein. She was one of the greatest literary innovators of the modern period, and some critics have suggested that she adopted her innovative style at least in part in order to be able to write about lesbianism safely and without censorship. Edmund Wilson suggested as much in 1951, although he retracted his theory at a later date. It is only with the advent of more recent *lesbian* writing, however, that the relationship between the two women is foregrounded (Faderman 1981, Rule 1975, Souhami 1991), and I am unaware of any critical attempt to assess Stein and Toklas as an authorial partnership.[11]

That Toklas typed and prepared Stein's work for publication is perfectly clear, what is less clear is the complexity present but hidden in their collaboration and perhaps implied by Stein's deflected autobiographical subject. Jane Rule (1975) suggests that the work may have been a collaboration between the two women, or even that they 'reversed roles' in writing it, with Stein typing to Toklas' dictation.

The question of collaboration is possibly of particular relevance to lesbian writing. Another famous instance is that of Michael Field, the *nom de plume* and shared persona of Katherine Bradley and Edith Cooper, 'poets and lovers from 1870 to 1913' (White 1992). Bradley and Cooper, who were aunt and niece, published jointly authored poetry (including a volume 'restoring' and extending Sappho's writings) under the name of Michael Field and appear to have been quite self-consciously lesbian (though see White's essay for a discussion of the difficulties in interpreting this 'lesbian'). They also left volumes of a journal, with instructions that they were to be opened and published at the end of 1929. Such collaborations, whether overt like theirs or suspected, like Stein's and Toklas', offer intriguing new perspectives on authorial identity and the strategies adopted by women writers, particularly lesbians.

More recently, Suniti Namjoshi and Gillian Hanscombe, lovers and poets, have chosen to publish their work jointly without distinguishing who wrote which poems (*Flesh and Paper*, 1986). This is presented by them as a specifically lesbian strategy: 'we lesbians, millions of us, now have a new understanding. We can speak in public. That means we can take the central "I" and "you" and "we" of the language of lyric poetry to mean ourselves, without compromise' (Namjoshi and Hanscombe 1986). By erasing the distinction between the two authorial 'I's, the erasure both of the barrier between writer and reader and of the distinguishing and distinctive binary of heterosexual difference (one male, one female) is made overt; as indeed is the erasure of the barrier of race/ethnicity, since Namjoshi is Indian and Black, and Hanscombe is Australian and white. Thus, textual practice becomes both a metaphor and enactment of a radical political goal.

Gertrude Stein, of all writers, had perhaps the most apt and perceptive critique of the relationship between art and reality, especially in the context of autobiography, where her insights cut decisively through the more portentious autobiographical navel-gazing of her male contemporary, Joyce. The last word on the subject may delightfully be left to Stein herself:

> And identity is funny being yourself is funny as you
> are never yourself to yourself except as you remember
> yourself and then of course you do not believe
> yourself. That is really the trouble with an
> autobiography you do not of course you do not really
> believe yourself why should you, you know so well so
> very well that it is not yourself, it could not be
> yourself because you cannot remember right and if
> you do remember right it does not sound right and of
> course it does not sound right because it is not right.
> You are of course never yourself.
>
> (extract from *Everybody's Autobiography*, in Souhami 1991)

DAPHNE 'NOT A LESBIAN' DU MAURIER AND THE BOY IN HER BOX

Homophobia shapes the ability and willingess of all lesbians, including those who write, to name themselves lesbian, as well as informing the content, form and genres used by lesbian authors. Bonnie Zimmerman identifies 'coming out stories, romances and utopias' as the staple forms of lesbian fiction (Zimmerman 1992a), and it is not hard to see the part played by these forms in making it possible to read oneself as a lesbian self against the grain of a heterosexist culture. The significance of writing to women's ability to name themselves 'lesbian' is crucial, as the case of Daphne du Maurier shows. But looking at lesbian questions, such as the life of du Maurier, without 'lesbian antennae' is problematic, as the recent biography of du Maurier indicates.

With the publication of Margaret Forster's biography (1993), du Maurier's sexual relationship with actress Gertrude Lawrence and her desperate unrequited passion for Ellen Doubleday have become public knowledge. She was clearly aware of being different from childhood. She wrote to Ellen of 'never being a little girl. Always being a little boy. And growing up with a boy's mind and a boy's heart . . . so that at 18 this half-breed fell in love, as a boy would' (Forster 1993: 222). She writes in other letters of locking 'the boy' up in a box, refers to that part of her self as 'my Jack-in-the-box' and describes herself at her first sight of Ellen Doubleday as 'a boy of 18 all over again with nervous hands and a beating heart, incurably romantic and wanting to throw a cloak before his lady's feet' (ibid.: 221). She had code words for homosexual feelings, which she called 'Venetian', and heterosexuality, which she called 'Cairo', complaining that she found 'Cairo' boring and unmoving and expressing her grief and frustration to Ellen that 'there will never be Venice with you'.

Yet all this, which reads now like a woman aware of and accepting her lesbianism, co-exists with bitter hostility towards lesbians. She wrote to Ellen that she would throw herself in the Hudson River if Ellen thought she was 'just one more Venetian wanting to make a pass', refusing 'to be classed with that gang' (ibid.: 231), and was, heart-breakingly, scared to love her son Kits too much, not wanting to 'turn him into a homo' (ibid.: 248). A still more explicit letter to Ellen vows 'by God and by Christ if anyone should call that sort of love by that unattractive word that begins with "L", I'd tear their guts out' (ibid.: 223).

Her biographer, Forster, leaves this remarkable set of contradictions to stand, unwilling or unable to make sense of them. Yet a critical lesbian reading offers much of interest, not only to lesbians but to anyone interested in the dynamics of the relationship between the sexual, the social and the textual. Du Maurier was not at all upset by, ashamed of or unwilling to admit her desire for women or her unin-volvement with heterosex. So *what* was she disavowing when she so violently disassociated herself from 'that unattractive word that begins with "L"'? A lesbian reading of her novel *Rebecca* gives us a clue, for the dead Rebecca's dreadful secret is precisely that she was a lesbian (Wings 1992b).[12] Rebecca's deviant sexuality is a secret *so* dreadful that, both in the eyes of the reader and in the eyes of his second wife, it justifies Maxim de Winter murdering her. His second wife's response, and it is one which we are directed by the narrative to share, is pity for her murderous husband. To be a lesbian, we are told, is a far worse crime than murder! To find out why du Maurier thought this, when she herself was quite clearly (to our eyes at least) a lesbian, requires an understanding of what 'lesbian' meant to her. What meanings of the 'unattractive word that begins with "L"' were available for her consumption in the literature, popular culture and social attitudes of her day? How did she *read* 'lesbian' in such a way as to make it impossible for her to *live* lesbian or *write* 'lesbian' as anything other than abhorrent? These are questions awaiting a lesbian biography of du Maurier; they are also questions which take us right to the heart of current literary theory. The active making-sense which is reading, the multiple and often competing possible readings of any text, the contingency of the sense embedded in the textual, the mutually *constitutive* relation of the textual and the social – all these are foregrounded in a peculiarly apt and vivid way by the complex nuances of du Maurier's personal, textual and dominant cultural 'lesbians'.

DANGEROUS TO KNOW – WRITING AND TEACHING 'LESBIAN'

It is easy to forget just how recent and how local has been the current (limited) freedom enjoyed by (some) lesbians. Gertrude Stein was forced to obscure her lesbianism to evade the censor; that Jeanette Winterson is able to be quite open about her sexuality does not mean that everything is now fine and dandy for lesbian writers and writing, nor does it retrospectively eradicate the fear and danger of writing as a lesbian even a decade ago. As recently as 1988, several contributors to Christine McEwan's collection of lesbian poetry *Naming the Waves* felt it necessary to write under a *nom de plume* or to remain anonymous, and Jane Rule very nearly lost her job as university lecturer after the 1964 publication of her lesbian romance *Desert of the Heart* (Rule 1975). Rule's own collection of lesbian criticism, *Lesbian Images*, the first book of its kind to be published, went out of print two years after publication. The publisher's note which opens the 1984 Crossing Press reprint comments, 'neither the author's growing literary reputation, nor the book's critical success in the media, nor the profitability of its sales, nor the supportive climate of a burgeoning lesbian feminist movement kept *Lesbian Images* on the bookshelves'.

If the 'burgeoning lesbian feminist movement' could not prevent the eradication of lesbian writing and scholarship it did make it possible for (some) women to acknowledge their lesbianism publicly for the first time. Rosemary Manning, for example, having been a writer all her life, was unable to come out as a lesbian until her seventies. The first chapter of her writer's autobiography details the slow process which enabled her to make sense of her lesbian identity over the course of a lifetime. 'When I was in my forties I at last acknowledged the truth to myself. Thirty years later, I proclaimed it' (Manning 1987). There is no other human experience comparable to this. To go through the first forty years of life with one's full self unacknowledged, and to then have to keep that self-knowledge secret until old age is a journey quite beyond the experience or understanding of most.

Nor are the pains and difficulties of writing as a lesbian safely in the pre-feminist past. The social penalties of being a lesbian have not gone away; the incomprehension, belittling and erasures of lesbian writing have not stopped. In Betsy Warland's (1991) collection of accounts by lesbian writers about what being a lesbian writer means, the contributors – and the list includes many established and respected names – speak of having to deal with pain, isolation, mistrust, misunderstanding, fear or straightforward homophobia. Minnie Bruce Pratt's account is both poignant and typical:

A flash of doubt, though I didn't change anything I was saying or reading, a flashback on other moments when I opened my mouth and *lesbian* came out in one form or another; and I feared the blow. As if my word might vapourize my children, my mother, the person offering me a job I might need, might obliterate me and my lover in a public place. The power of my own word turned against me.

(in Warland 1991: 27)

How can one little word have so much power? The thing which a lesbian reading can never let go of is that this power has been literal. The word 'lesbian' *has done all the things which the writer fears it will do.* Being lesbian has cost women their children, their families, their jobs, their lovers and their lives. We are not, when we speak or write about 'lesbian oppression' talking about being excluded from polite society. We are talking clear and present danger. The 'lesbian' which lesbian writers write and which lesbian readers read is not only the essential raw material of lesbian becoming on an individual level, it is also an oppositional lesbian cultural presence in the world. 'Lesbian' is a word given vociferous meaning by homophobia – in the gutter press, in medical discourse, in legislation, in sensationalist popular culture, in the variously vicious doctrines of fundamentalist religion. The 'lesbian' written and read *by* lesbians challenges that vociferousness. As Luz Maria

Umpierre writes 'I write because writing is the only tool I have to maintain my sanity in a world and country that have grown increasingly insane and insensitive to difference. . . . In writing I find a developing identity. In writing I can define our story' (in Warland 1991).

TEACHING LESBIAN LITERATURE

It is not enough to write and read 'lesbian'. Lesbian critical commentary is as essential to lesbian literature as to any other genre. Indeed, it is obvious from what has been discussed in this chapter that lesbian literary scholarship is of very real importance to the lesbian 'community', to lesbian existence. So how does lesbian literature get taught? It is still almost exclusively left to lesbians to teach lesbian literature, and if writing or reading as a lesbian have been difficult, teaching lesbian literature has been next to impossible. Mainstream society is saturated with homophobic anxiety, an anxiety which finds peculiar expression in the belief that homosexuals are child molesters out to 'convert' the young (Bulkin 1981), so teaching openly *as* a lesbian or *about* lesbian issues or texts is seldom possible in a school context. Teaching lesbian- (and/or gay) themed literature in school English programmes remains dangerous and difficult in the context of increasingly hostile legislation in both the USA and the UK,[13] despite powerful argument that this is precisely when and where such teaching *should* take place (Harris 1990).

Even teachers working in universities or colleges find that teaching lesbian literature makes their professional lives difficult (see papers in Cruikshank 1982) and their relationship with their students fraught (Bulkin 1981). One factor which distinguishes this kind of teaching from teaching about other difficult issues is the question of contamination-by-association. If you presume to offer your students lesbian literature you must be lesbian – an assumption with complex implications for both lesbian and non-lesbian teachers – and if you are 'out' as a lesbian teacher, then your private life is up for grabs: 'students felt quite free to ask personal questions designed to fill in the gaps in their knowledge: about my coming out, my daughter, lesbian sexuality and relationships, my parents' reaction to my lesbianism' (Bulkin 1981).

LESBIAN CRITICISM – DEFINED OUT OF EXISTENCE?

Lesbian literary criticism, of which there is a large and steadily growing body, ranges from book reviews in lesbian and gay magazines to highly theoretical commentary within the academy. As far as range goes, lesbian lit. crit. is little different from the non-lesbian variety. The positioning of the lesbian critic in relation to the lesbian 'community' and to hegemonic narratives of gender and sexuality, however, gives rise to a unique kind of criticism, a criticism which itself operates to construct a variety of lesbianisms. And such lesbianisms become increasingly difficult for a flesh-and-blood lesbian to inhabit, let alone for a lesbian writer/reader to make use of in any unproblematically developmental way. Almost all collections of lesbian criticism begin by addressing what Chris Weedon calls 'the primary problem of identifying lesbian texts' (Weedon 1987: 158). In this, lesbian criticism has an additional problem to reckon with. Not only must it be decided whether the 'lesbian-ness' of a text is located in its author, its content, its writing or its reading(s), it must also be decided what, for the purposes of the critical task, lesbian-ness *is*. The interrogation/deconstruction of 'lesbian' is an intrinsic part of lesbian literary studies.

Sally Munt suggests that deconstruction is something which lesbians readers are, by their very nature, good at: 'Lesbians are particularly adept at deconstruction, patiently reading between the lines, from the margins, inhabiting the text of dominant heterosexuality even as we undo it, undermine it and construct our own destabilising images' (Munt 1992: xiii), and this is certainly a compelling argument. However, existing as she does in the hinterland of heterosexist denial, it is particularly devastating for a lesbian to erase 'lesbian' textually. Claudie Lesselier writes of 'the tension between, on the one hand, *claiming a category* by giving it another meaning and, on the other hand, *subverting the whole system of categorization*' (Lesselier 1987, in Meese 1992). Yet this is the process which most lesbian critics agree is *the* privileged marker of the lesbian-ness of texts.

Lesbian criticism constructs a specifically textual 'lesbian' who has no straightforward linear relationship to the 'social' or 'psychological' lesbian we have been discussing. This lesbian *is* a textual creature, whose political importance derives from her disruptive and disobedient presence within/against the master narrative of the heteropatriarchy. Monique Wittig, whose book *The Lesbian Body* is probably the most important lesbian text yet written and whose bold claim is that 'lesbians are not women' (Wittig 1981), writes (in explanation of her own textual practice):

> The *j/e* with a bar in *The Lesbian Body* is not an *I* destroyed. It is an *I* become so powerful that it can attack the order of heterosexuality in

texts and assault so-called love, the heroes of love, and lesbianize them, lesbianize the symbols, lesbianize the gods and godesses, lesbianize men and women.

(Wittig 1985, in Farwell 1992)[14]

This textual lesbian then, this *j/e*, functions to disrupt heterpolarity, to contaminate the certainties of the hegemonic narrative (certainties such as 'men' and 'women'), and this is certainly the understanding shared by many lesbian critics and writers. For Bonnie Zimmerman one of the radical aspects of lesbian literature is that, unlike woman-centred hetero-sexual feminist literature, 'a lesbian text places men firmly at the margins of the story' (Zimmerman 1992). The difficulty with this seems to me obvious: to what extent may a work such as Gertrude Stein's *Autobiography of Alice B. Toklas* be said to 'place men firmly at the margins of the story'? Furthermore, defining lesbian texts in relation to their treatment of men simply reinforces the androcentrism and phallo-gocentrism which feminists criticise in literature.

Another approach is to claim for lesbians a *higher* nature than the merely heterosexual. For novelist Bertha Harris, according to Zimmer-man, '"lesbian" is a more profoundly human definition than "woman" because it disrupts the inevitable connection between sex and reproduc-tion' (Zimmerman 1992: 44). Again, this is fraught with problems, not least of which is the failure of feminists to theorise motherhood ade-quately. *Why* is it 'more profoundly human' to 'disrupt the inevitable connection between sex and reproduction', and in what way (if at all) does 'lesbian' disrupt this connection more radically than 'contraceptive pill'?

Having cynically questioned the facility with which 'lesbian' is con-structed as privileged radical other *per se*, it is nevertheless true to say that lesbian-ness is perhaps the only way of exposing and challenging the heteropolarity of the master narrative of Western culture. Lesbian writing exposes the difficulty for non-lesbian women of escaping entirely their identification with men (Bennett 1992, Parker 1992, Weedon 1987). Alice Parker suggests that 'any woman who identifies with men labours under a terrific historical burden of male fantasy',[15] and a lesbian writing/reading makes this perfectly clear. She further suggests that 'lesbian love is a discourse that disrupts or radically interrogates all of the authorising codes of our culture' (Parker 1992: 319).

While it is certainly true that lesbian texts/the textual lesbian functions in this disruptive way (although 'real' lesbians do not see discursive disruption as their *raison d'être*), Bonnie Zimmerman alerts us to the dangers inherent in privileging 'lesbian' in this way. Whilst agreeing that 'lesbian' functions as a radical signifier she warns against privileging lesbian-as-radical-sign over other excluded and marginal positions, arguing instead that we should adopt Teresa de Lauretis' notion of the 'eccentric subject', 'the subject who exists across boundaries and in a marginal or tangential relation to the white, Western, middle-class male centre' (Zimmerman 1992b).

CONCLUSION

Literature, then, is essential to lesbians, enabling a construction of lesbian subjectivity and of a sexual and social identity. Lesbian-ness is important to literary studies, enabling a recognition of and challenge to the heterosexist and homophobic nature of the established canon and introducing a necessary eccentric perspective from which may be 'read' the hegemonic structures and relations of the heteropatriarchy as they impact on and inflect the production and consumption of literary texts. Yet these two processes exist in mutual conflict: the usefulness of lesbian fiction (Zimmerman 1992a) in constructing a 'lesbian' reader is undermined by the usefulness of the lesbian-as-privileged-other to the project of deconstructing gender/erotic categories altogether. This apparent contradiction is, I would suggest, not as direct or as straightforwardly binary as it appears. If, as Zimmerman suggests, 'lesbian culture is like a philosophical or religious system that provides its adherents with a way of viewing the world anew' (ibid.: 14), then flexibility, the contingency of 'identity' and the multiple positionings of 'lesbian' in relation to culture, self and the erotic may easily be a structuring force in that 'system'. As such, 'lesbian' may become one of the nicest ways to 'be' in postmodernity. Indeed, Munt suggests that lesbian culture represents the ideal of postmodernism – unlike feminism, which she sees as anti-postmodern (Munt 1992: 33–4). Or, to cite Marilyn Farwell, 'lesbian' may be understood not as a kind of person, but as a cultural and textual position: 'Ahistoricism and essentialism are the central problems which have plagued the attempt to define lesbian metaphorically. I believe that some of these problems are eliminated when one speaks of lesbian as a space rather than as an essence' (Farwell 1992).

For 'lesbian' to be a space (and I am struck between the cultural critical notion of lesbian-as-space and Mary McIntosh's sociological notion of the homosexual role) is not only a solution to the problem of lesbian subjectivity, it is also an important way forward for lesbian feminism. For a space called 'lesbian' is available for *any* woman to move into, to inhabit. Just as a space called 'Black' becomes a potential 'reading site' for *all* readers. As Zimmerman reminds us:

> The lesbian is one, but only one, embodiment of this eccentric subject, with her own peculiarities, her own histories, her own textual strategies, and her own specific disruptive practices. One future direction for lesbian criticism, then, lies in investigating the specificity of the lesbian subject, or subjects.
>
> (Zimmerman 1992b: 7)

And this, I believe, is finally what lesbian literary studies is 'about' – developing a 'lesbian space' from which any reader, whether 'really' lesbian or not, may read any text. The critical, social and political potential of such readings would be truly radical.

NOTES

1 As it does for gay men too, of course, but gay male scholarship is not yet as finely tuned to gender sensitivity as is lesbian scholarship. An ironic example of this is Sedgwick's work (1985, 1991), which, although described by her as feminist, demonstrates a strange opacity towards gender issues as integral to heterosexism (Castle 1992).

2 I have put 'gay' in what Sedgwick calls 'scare quotes' to indicate that it is, of course, far from unproblematic to think of Shakespeare, Plato or even Proust as gay . . . male same-sex eroticism carrying such shifting meanings across even tiny distances in time and space as to make the act of claiming these three writers (or any writer not of the post-Stonewall industrialised and urban West) as gay an act of semantic colonialism indistinct from the ethocentrism and androcentrism we quite rightly reject in mainstream scholarship. Nevertheless, they have all left ample evidence of sexual engagement with members of their own sex.

3 But see the above note regarding the fluidity of sexual nomenclature.

4 Not, of course, all lesbian and gay criticism. Recent collections (I am thinking of Bristow 1992, Fuss 1991 or Plummer 1992) have achieved a relatively equitable balance between gay male and lesbian theory.

5 Of course, just because it is intellectually absurd does not mean it no longer happens! The ideological and partial nature of the academy is brought into sharp focus by its continued stubborn adherence to the intellectually moribund practices of racism, sexism and heterosexism, which have been concealed so long by and within its unchallenged (because so successfully exclusive) supremacy.

6 . . . and with current advances in digitalising photographic imagery it is uncertain how much longer a photograph will be acceptable documentary evidence of anything, let alone something as generally unlikely as the existence of lesbians!

7 Passing women did, of course, sometimes pass as men precisely in order to deal with sexism, but although their number is probably greater than we suspect or shall ever know, this remains an uncommon response to patriarchal power.

8 By using the phrase 'growing up lesbian' here, I am not meaning to imply that lesbians are born not made, nor that women's sexual orientation/ preference is unchanging (see pp. 29–49).

9 Even the mayonnaise jar sitting in my fridge as I write is adorned with a scene depicting a heterosexual couple having a romantic (mayonnaise-saturated) picnic in the country. And they call *us* blatant . . .

10 She is quoting Hortense Spillers' essay 'Interstices – a small drama of words' (in Vance 1984).

11 Still, other silences replace the ruptured silence surrounding their lesbianism. Diana Souhami, for example, whose book *Gertrude and Alice* (1991) takes as its subject their life partnership, referred several times during a talk she delivered during Feminist Book Festival 1993 to their 'typical Christian marriage'. Stein and Toklas were, in fact, Jews! I suspect there is interesting work to be done on Toklas as 'Jewish momma'.

12 Mary Wings, writer of popular lesbian thrillers, in fact modelled her 1992 novel *Divine Victim* on a lesbian re-telling of the plot of *Rebecca*; her paper at the York conference included a witty exposé of the signifiers of lesbianism embedded in the Hollywood film version of *Rebecca*.

13 Though not, of course, in all other European countries! Sweden, Holland and Denmark, for example, demonstrate a far more enlightened approach to teaching lesbian and gay issues in schools.

14 It is interesting to note that Farwell is citing Wittig here to support her argument concerning a lesbian pulp fantasy novel, *The Mists of Avalon* (Bradley 1982). Using theoretical 'big guns' such as Wittig to discuss pulp fiction is an important indicator of the transgressive approach to genre status which is so much a part of lesbian criticism and which makes lesbian-ness so troubling a presence in literary studies.

15 There are, of course, many lesbian writers who make quite free with the accusation that other lesbians (especially 'sex radical' or SM lesbians) are 'male-identified', and the construction of lesbians as *not* identifying with men becomes a very moot point when considering the lesbian-and-gay community and all the fruitful collaborations there have been and continue to be between homosexual women and men. However, I think the point remains, since it is about the pervasive pressures on women who have sex with men (and I include bisexual women here) to please men.

Chapter 7

Lesbians studying culture
Studying lesbian culture

Art is a major battleground in the struggle for self-determination – for gay people even more than for others, because, unique among subgroups, we are not born into our own culture.

(Saslow 1978)

She needs warm compresses for her eyes if nowhere else, due to the dearth of Lesbian films and the need to do a salvage job on Supergirl.

(Lahire 1987)

[A]rt made by and for heterosexuals with little thought of homosexuality looks very different if seen from a lesbian perspective.

(Richards 1990)

LESBIAN LOOKING/HEARING/SPEAKING

As with other fields within lesbian studies, lesbian cultural studies has a dual focus; deploying what might be thought of as the academic gaze both from the position 'cultural studies' towards 'lesbian' and simultaneously from the position 'lesbian' towards 'culture' and, indeed, 'cultural studies' itself. One imperative is to identify and critique the location of 'lesbian' among the activities of textual productivity. Another is to engage with the lesbian-ness of 'lesbian' culture and with the processes and products which go to make up that culture. Suffice it to say that these two projects are neither discrete nor mutually exclusive.

It is impossible to outline 'lesbian cultural studies' in one chapter. This chapter glances briefly at the visual arts (painting, photography, sculpture, drawing, etc.) and the time-based media (film, television, video, music, theatre, dance). I am unhappy not to have been able to look in more detail at theatre, performance art, dance and the broadcast media. Although there is material available on some of these (Goodman

1993, Griffin 1993, Hamer and Budge 1994), on others there is at best a fragmentary body of work. The lesbian perspective on dance, for example, is embryonic.

Lesbian cultural production encompasses both 'high' and 'popular' forms and its values do not necessarily (or even commonly) coincide with those of traditional academic criticism. In this and in its deviant readings of non-lesbian texts, lesbian culture is in some sense paradigmatically postmodern. This is interesting not only to a study of 'lesbian culture' – meaning the loose and amorphous homeland of the imaginary for lesbian women, constructed by means of shared (and disputed) signs and texts – but also to a study of culture itself and its relation to hegemony, group/personal identity and truth-hierarchies. As with lesbian literary studies and its problematising of 'the canon', the partial and political nature of mainstream criticism is exposed by a set of practices which coalesces around an entirely different set of values.

A BRUSH WITH LESBIANS: PAINTING

Any lesbian critique of painting must begin with feminist work in this field. Feminists have claimed that the 'gaze' of Western art is male, that women are commodified and fetishised through and by that gaze and the practices it informs (Mulvey 1972), and that women's art is suppressed through sexist institutional practices, including male-dominated art schools and funding bodies which ignore the existence of women. The feminist critique locates gender relations in the 'relationship between mark-making and the social construction of femininity' (Chadwick 1990: 350). In the USA, the group Guerrilla Girls has since the late 1980s been carrying out poster campaigns protesting the sexism and racism in the commercial art world. Their tactics have been appropriated by a similar group in Britain, Fanny Adam, which has received Arts Council Funding for some of its work. Such campaigns, which in true postmodern parodic style risk segueing from political statement into radical chic, do serve to foreground issues of gender in the Art establishment.

Yet a lesbian perspective has been largely absent from all this industriousness; indeed, feminist commentary risks reifying heterosexuality precisely because of its foundational critique of gender. Important feminist theorists and historians of the visual arts such as Linda Nochlin, Griselda Pollock, Whitney Chadwick or Laura Mulvey leave no space for a lesbian gaze in their analyses.

The lesbian is as phantasmically present-as-absence in feminist art criticism as she is anywhere. For example, Pollock's piece 'Screening the seventies: sexuality and representation' is about *heterosexuality* and representation. At one point Pollock discusses Yves Lomax's 'Open rings and partial lines', a 'protest against the binary oppositions which underpin the heterosexist regime of sexual difference' (Pollock 1988: 175). This is surely of great significance to Pollock's exploration of feminist attempts to subvert the positioning of women within art as always already the object of the male (erotic/posessive) gaze. Yet the essay seamlessly passes over the implications of a lesbian (desiring) gaze or the lesbian refusal of the male gaze, thus reinforcing what Pollock seeks to challenge.

Feminist critics can be extraordinarily wilful in their refusal to see that lesbians exist. Joanne Issack has this to say in reference to Mary Kelly's notorious transformation of Freudian theory into art in 'Post Partum Document (PPD)' and her later work, 'Interim':

> If the mother who knows sexual pleasure, the subject of Mary Kelly's *PPD* is the most severely repressed 'feminine' figure in Western culture, then the middle-aged woman runs a close second. For Lacan the assumption of an image occasions desire, the middle age marks the occasion of the loss of that assumed image, of not being the object of man's desire, of being out of sync with how you look, of alienation from your image.
>
> (Issack 1985: 5)

It may well be true that, for a *heterosexual* woman, not being 'the object of man's desire' makes you 'out of sync with how you look', but in what way could that possibly be true for lesbian women? In a familiar vanishing, both the lesbian and the specificity of women's oppression within heterosexuality are made not-there. Issack's silence ensures that the lesbian joins the sexual mother as the most 'severely repressed "feminine" figure in Western culture', while neither artist nor critic take into account the social control of the lesbian, whose unfitness to mother is located precisely in the sexualisation of her lesbian-ness.

A major unrecognised problem for mainstream feminist art theory is that it relies on an absolute presumption of heterobinary dynamics. Linda Nochlin, agreeing with Laura Mulvey, writes:

> [T]here are two choices open to the woman spectator: either to take the place of the male or to accept the position of male created seductive passivity and the questionable pleasure of masochism – lack of power to the nth degree.
>
> (Nochlin 1989: 30)

There two choices refuse the possibility of *lesbian* looking and, by that refusal, reify and reproduce the heterosexual dynamic which Mulvey and Nochlin wish to undo. In fact, recognising a queer presence destabilises the feminist construction of Western Art as heterosexual power play. It would be hard to suggest a field of human activity where there was a more pronounced queer presence – has there ever been a gay Michelangelo? The fact that for every heterosexual Renoir, busy painting (women) with his prick there is a Michelangelo, a Leonardo, a Botticelli, a Caravaggio or a Hockney should trouble the heterosexual/heterosexist presumptions of straight feminist criticism and should point to more specific questions – questions such as why the male nude is so widely subsumed within the category 'homoerotic', while to regard the female nude in this light never seems to occur to anyone: surely this in itself constitutes an important unseen insight into the androcentricity of the art-critical apparatus?

No one would suggest that Botticelli's 'Birth of Venus' or (even) the pseudo-lesbian soft porn of Courbet's 'Sleep' are *intended* to provoke lesbian desire. Yet foregrounding the issue of spectatorship makes possible an exploration of disobedient lesbian consumption of supposedly heterosexual marks. That this has not happened to any significant degree has, I suggest, made it difficult for feminist art criticism/theory to move forward. Taking 'the place of the male' is *not* the same as taking a lesbian position, and there are important issues for feminism in the exploration of this difference – a difference in which may be located the specifics of male power.

The erasure of lesbian-ness from feminist art criticism occasionally leads to hilariously innocent readings. In 1974 Linda Benglis, an established artist, published a photograph of herself in *Artforum*, nude and oiled, sporting a pair of cool shades and a larger-than-life[1] dildo. Yet the lesbian potential of this image went unremarked upon, even by the artist herself: 'Benglis intended it as "the ultimate mockery of the pinup and the macho" (and the dildo image is a bizarre blend of the two)' (Tickner 1987: 248). I find it difficult to comprehend the entrenched heterosexism which refuses to glimpse any suggestion of lesbian possibility in the image of a naked woman wielding a dildo. A case of frantically re-repressing the returned repressed? Additionally, I find it cause for concern that a heterosexual woman may use a dildo to 'mock the pinup and the macho' and be supported in her actions by feminist commentators, while lesbian women's use of dildos is condemned as an obedient and reactionary imitation of male power (Jeffreys 1990, Loulan 1987).

There have been and continue to be successful lesbian painters. Feminists have tended to marginalise the significance of this presence, a strange oversight when one of their central (albeit unrecognised) themes has been the limitations on women's creative productivity imposed by heterosexuality (Greer 1979). The feminist treatment of Rosa Bonheur is a case in point (see pp. 55–6). Germaine Greer is unwilling to grant Bonheur's relationship with Natalie Micas unambiguously lesbian status: 'However much sex there was in their relationship, there was no dearth of love' (Greer 1979: 59). She is also unable to conceive of Bonheur's possible lesbianism as anything other than 'fear of the marauding activities of heterosexual men' (ibid.: 57), and only too happy to dismiss Micas as 'a rather ridiculous personage in many ways, with her pretensions to medical and veterinary knowledge', a put-down which echoes rather unpleasantly the typical dismissal of women by male writers. This is considerably better than Nochlin's account of Bonheur, however, which focuses entirely on 'the struggle between traditional history painting . . . and genre painting' and the economic conditions of the art industry in the nineteenth century. 'The success of Rosa Bonheur', she writes, 'firmly establishes the role of institutions, and institutional change, as a necessary, if not a sufficient, cause of achievement in art' (Nochlin 1989: 170). Although this statement forms part of the then new materialist approach to art criticism, which located art in systems of production rather than in individual genius, it fails to recognise the institutional effect of heterosexuality.[2] Writers such as Faderman (1991) identify the economic changes which followed the Industrial Revolution as necessary to and catalytic of modern lesbian identities and lifestyles. It is surely extremely important for a feminist theory and history of art to explore these intersecting currents of economics and sexuality rather than to ignore them.

The lesbian seeking to evaluate the lesbian-ness of Western Art, or even to make a list of known lesbian artists, is faced with a feminist art critical practice which is more profoundly heterosexist than the art it seeks to criticise and with a lesbian and gay studies which demonstrates little interest in lesbians, being inevitably dominated by men. It is at times like this that lesbian chutzpah, in the shape of lesbian-affirmative 'fun' publications such as Dell Richards *Lesbian Lists* (1990), comes to the rescue. Although light in tone and with no academic pretensions, such books offer a useful starting point for lesbian students. Alongside a list of '12 on-screen kisses and slow dances' may be found '9 lesbian artists' and '6 lesbian photographers of the past'. When academic books do not list 'lesbian' in their index the importance of such community-affirmative publications becomes immense!

Starting with this fragile thread in our hands, it is possible to enter the labyrinth of denial and erasure to bring Anna Klumpke, Mary Edmonia Lewis, Harriet Hosmer, Marie Laurencin and Romaine Brooks to the light of day (although Gluck would remain buried), and much work remains to be done on the lives and work of these women and on the meaning of their sexuality.

LESBIANS IN ART: WHAT DO WE MEAN?

Research also waits to be done on the meaning(s) of 'lesbian' in the work of painters such as Frida Kahlo or Tamara de Lempicka. There could not be two more different women. Kahlo was committed to the Mexican Revolution and she once took Trotsky as her lover. Lempicka was a baroness, a refugee from the Russian Revolution and decadent doyenne of Paris and New York society. Both were apparently bisexual, but desire for women is given very different meanings in their work.

For de Lempicka, an Art Deco painter who flirted with cubism and surrealism, lesbian love becomes an integral part of the decadent lasciviousness (in her life as much as her art) for which she was nicknamed 'a perverse Ingres'(Neret 1992, Phillips 1987). De Lempicka's 'lesbian' has much in common with the 'lesbian' of Baudelaire, Louys or Renée Vivien – a lost creature, tortured with insatiable lusts, heavy eyed with lack of sleep and sexual over-indulgence – and she painted many such creatures.

Kahlo painted mostly self-portraits, and only a few lesbian images are to be found in her *oeuvre* (in 'What I saw in the water' [1938] and 'Two nudes in the wood' [1939], for example). Much of her work is concerned with her own physical pain (she was left permanently disabled by an horrific street car accident when she was 18) and by the emotional pain caused by the infidelities of her husband, mural painter Diego Rivera. Yet she certainly had passionate affairs with women (Poniatowska and Stellweg 1992), and among the facets of identity which she confronted in her work and in her life was her 'butch' side. She was often photographed wearing men's clothing, and a famous painting, 'Self-portrait with cropped hair', shows her in a man's suit, surrounded by locks of hair, having shorn her head. The words of a popular song are painted above: 'Mira que si te fue por il pelo, Ahora que estas pelon, ya no te quiero' ('I loved you for your hair, now that you have cut your hair, I do not love you'). Laura Mulvey and Peter Wollen interpret this painting in Freudian terms, claiming that it represents for Kahlo a 'leap from the interior pain caused by her love for Diego to the wound left on the female body by castration' (Mulvey 1989: 91).

A lesbian commentator might note that it was not her love but Diego's betrayal which caused her pain,[3] and that this painting follows on very interestingly from the two lesbian images found in paintings of 1938 and 1939. Moreover, the Frida of this self-portrait is firmly placed on the canvas, upright on a sturdy chair, gazing at the viewer with what looks more like unapologetic defiance than grief. This is in marked contrast to many other self-portraits, which depict Kahlo as a baby, a wounded deer, a tearful and broken victim, the tiny wife of a larger-than-life Diego. Given that Frida developed such a direct and rich vocabulary with which to show her pain and vulnerability, I suggest that we trust her presentation of strength and solidity in 'Self-portrait with cropped hair'. This is not a woman mourning her lack of a penis but a strong woman constructing self-reliance out of her refusal of femininity.

Two such contrasting painters, two such different sets of meaning for 'lesbian'. Much remains to be gleaned from a lesbian study of de Lempicka and Kahlo (and many others): their positioning relative to the political struggles around them, the positioning of 'lesbian' in relation to those same struggles, their response to the 'lesbian' of their time and place, the meaning which their 'lesbian' images hold for a lesbian spectator today, the significance of the lesbian relationships they both had. By such inquiry our understanding of the complex relationships among sexuality, sexual identity, politics, historical moment, class, culture/ethnicity, gender and art begin to develop a tighter focus, a stronger base. By refusing to make lesbian meanings we are restricted to a partial and politically static enterprise, forever seeing Kahlo in the shadow of Rivera, unable to comprehend de Lempicka's self-conscious perversity.

ALIVE ALIVE OH! LIVING LESBIAN ARTISTS

But it is to the work of living lesbian artists that we must turn if we want to focus on lesbians in postmodern culture and on the construction of lesbian-ness by and for lesbians. There are few out lesbian artists and their public profile is markedly different from that of gay male artists. There is no lesbian Hockney or Mapplethorpe. The marginalisation of sexual minorities around which queer politics is structured is a clearly inadequate explanation for this situation. But so, too, is a feminist perspective, which, while identifying the material consequences of compulsory heterosexuality as the primary reason why there have been no great women artists (Greer 1979, Nochlin 1989), fails to name it as such and has failed to theorise lesbian oppression within feminist art history.

While lesbian artists are confronted by the material obstacles common to most women, they labour under the added burden of *lesbian* oppression. Contemporary British lesbian painter Rachel Field is clear in her analysis of the intersections of gender and sexuality in the art world: 'Male homoerotica is sublimated throughout cultural history, reaffirming the phallocracy. It is dissipated throughout the mainstream because of the dominance and control of masculinity, whilst lesbians have remained anonymous' (Field 1990). She is equally clear about the failure of feminism to incorporate a lesbian perspective and about the complicity of feminists in lesbian oppression:

> Feminist art of the 1970s and early 1980s has been monopolized by heterosexual women. . . . Heterosexual women have used their art as a palliative to the male ego, seemingly to attack but always presenting themselves in relationship to men and never rejecting the privileges of heterosexuality. Heterosexual women artists have shown a fear of the 'aggressive and predatory' lesbian in a similar way to the rejection lesbians experienced in the Women's Liberation Movement in the early 1970s.
>
> (Field 1990: 115)

Field's response to the oppression she experiences in her daily life as a lesbian and to the inadequacy of straight feminist art is to paint her lesbian-ness. Colourful, witty and figurative, her art is, 'as much as art ever is, accessible, whilst promoting what to many will be an incomprehensible message' (ibid.: 118). The titles are an intrinsic part of the whole: 'Illegal on the street', a lyrical painting of one woman offering another a flower, shows the two frozen in the act of beginning a kiss. To a lesbian viewer this painting encodes powerfully the condition of living out one's deepest affections under surveillance, the countless kisses, embraces and other simple gestures of love which we are denied in a lifetime, the freezing of lesbian intimacy under the regime of compulsory heterosexuality. Heterosexual viewers, as Field has found, often refuse/fail to see her paintings: 'Rachel Field's paintings didn't really articulate for me anything about what it must feel like to be a lesbian' and 'her figures are almost without the attributes of sex' are comments from writers of two separate reviews in the *Women Artists Slide Library Journal* (Pearson 1989, Morris 1988, in Field 1990: 119). Field points out that 'both the female reviewers state clearly in the articles their heterosexuality and therefore their nonaffiliation with the sexuality I am portraying' (ibid.: 119).

Feminist art theory and criticism is clearly antagonistic to lesbians and lesbian-ness, while the malestream (including the gay malestream) merely 'includes lesbians out' in its continued marginalisation of all women's art. In response, groups such as the Lesbian Artists' Network[4] are starting to form, and hopefully such collective initiatives will enable the development of a strong body of lesbian work and lesbian criticism and commentary.

DRAWING THE LINE – CARTOONING AS A SUBVERSIVE ACTIVITY

It is no coincidence, I suggest, that many living lesbian artists are cartoonists. Cartooning is small scale, needs no vast studio, no expensive canvas, paints or stretchers, no public funding or commercial sponsorship, no entroit into the magic circle of galleries and exhibition space.[5] It is also a short-lived art form, ideal for political and social comment, and in this age of high-tech, low-cost printing and desk-top publishing, is cheap and easily accessible. In addition, humour can be both a sharp political weapon and the social glue of communities under seige – witness Jewish humour. There are many lesbian cartoonists, drawing regular strips for lesbian and gay magazines and newspapers, contributing to women's comics and low-tech 'zines such as *Shocking Pink* and its successor, *Bad Attitude*, publishing postcards, greetings cards, calendars and coffee-table humorous collections.

It is hard to overstate the importance of seemingly trite artefacts such as calendars and postcards in a hostile world. For the most part, lesbians are cultural scavengers, stealing from the fringes of the heterosexual master-text by a process of co-option, re-coding, reading against the grain and inverting/inventing meanings disobedient to authorial intent. So it is hugely significant to be able to purchase each year a calendar made for and by lesbians, which reflects lesbian interests and lesbian issues. And if it is humorous, so much the better. Alison Bechdel's 'Dykes to watch out for' calendars and annual cartoon collections, featuring the characters from her eponymous cartoon strip, are important lesbian artefacts, a source of pride and reassurance. We still exist, we've survived another year! In addition, Bechdel's light and certain touch enables her to deal with quite serious and often difficult issues. Collections such as Kate Charlesworth's *Exotic Species* (1984), characters such as Leigh Dunlap's Morgan Calabrese (1987, 1989) or Cath Jackson's Vera the Visible Lesbian (1984, 1986), or gag books like *The Lesbian Survival Manual* (Dicksion 1990) or *Cut-Outs and Cut-Ups* (Dean *et al.* 1989) strengthen the sense of lesbian community by poking gentle fun at it, bear witness to the quotidian mundanities of living in a hostile world and offer relief from the serious and dangerous business of being a dyke.

The comic-book formula has also been used effectively by, for example, the Hetrick-Martin Institute for the Protection of Lesbian and Gay Youth in New York, which publishes a series of narrative comic-books, *Tales of the Closet*, as part of its outreach work with young lesbians and gay men (Hetrick-Martin Institute 1988, 1989). Covering topics such as homophobic violence, health and relationships, the comic-books invite comment from readers and hope to provide a service for young lesbians and gay men who, as research repeatedly indicates, are among the most isolated and vulnerable groups in society (Comstock 1991, Herdt 1989).

Cartooning, like the pulp novels of the 1950s, has an importance to the lesbian community quite unlike its heterosexual equivalent. Yet neither feminist nor lesbian and gay cultural studies has paid lesbian (or gay) cartoonists much attention, with the notable exception of Tom of Finland, whose unmistakable and highly skilled 'dirty drawings' (his own description) played such a significant part in the reclaiming of masculinity by gay male culture (Hooven 1992).[6] Given the rise to respectability within cultural studies of the graphic novel and the comic-book, hopefully we will soon see at least a slim monograph on the significance of the cartoonist's art to lesbian politics!

DOC-PHOT AND EROT-PHOT? LESBIAN PHOTOGRAPHY

Contemporary Western culture is densely saturated with photographic images. This is as true of lesbian (and gay) culture as anywhere else: from the parodic radical trash photo-stories in local lesbian 'zines (for example, *Diversion* 1991) to the Lacanian hype of Della Grace's work in *New Formations* (Adams 1993), lesbian photography is a voluble presence. Yet, unsurprisingly, feminist histories of women photographers either make the briefest token mention of lesbian photographers (Williams 1987) or fail to mention them altogether (Fisher 1987), despite the fact that important woman photographers, such as Berenice Abbott and Alice Austen, were lesbian.

Photography, as Susan Sontag suggests, is 'a grammar and, even more importantly, an ethics of seeing' (Sontag 1977: 3). How, then, to ensure a lesbian syntax in that grammar, a lesbian ethics of seeing? If, as Sontag says, 'the most grandiose result of the photographic enterprise is to give us the sense that we can hold the whole world in our heads – as an anthology of images' (ibid.: 3), it is important that this cerebral anthology should not be condemned to unthinking heterobinarism.

How to say 'lesbian' in photography is perhaps the key problem. Because we are defined by/as our sexual selves, an unmistakable lesbian photographic image, and one resistant to heterosexist erasure, is obliged to present a sexualised 'lesbian' – or to depend upon extra-textual labelling/interpretation of the image, such as a caption saying the 'lesbian', which the photograph cannot. The alternative, to resort to cultural signifiers and codes such as labyris jewellery, shaved heads or black triangles, privileges the decoding abilities of a specifically situated lesbian viewer, excluding from the hermeneutic conversation those not so situated.

Self-consciously lesbian photography has tended to fall into two strands, the documentary and the sexual. The documentary has a long history. Both feminist and queer photographers have documented their communities and struggles. The documentary project of the gay community has gained a new edge and urgency with the documentation of the lives of people living with HIV (see Camerawork/The Photo Co-op 1989, Photographers and Friends United Against AIDS 1990). Such documentation has been mostly in the genre of social realism, recording the range of women's experiences in anthologies such as *Women See Women* (Wiesenfeld *et al.* 1976) or *Emergence* (Macadams 1977), or presenting a cast of lesbian and gay community figures such as *Positive Image* (Stewart 1985). Documenting the existence and struggles of lesbians remains an important political task. Brenda Prince, Mikki Ferrill, Della Grace and others continue to record key moments in lesbian lives: Gay Pride and Lesbian Strength marches, the day-to-day lives of lesbian mothers, the fight against Section 28. There has been a recent trend towards what might be called symbolic documentary, using set-dressing, staging, cut-and-paste and other techniques to represent the complex cultural and social factors which intersect in the site of resistance which is the queer body. Gay photographers like the late Rotimi Fani-Kayode and Alex Hirst have developed a fecund symbolic vocabulary with which to speak about being gay, as have lesbian photographers Tee Corinne, Ingrid Pollard, Jacqui Duckworth, the much mourned Tessa Boffin and others. Other axes of difference/oppression converge in the work of lesbians of colour, as they do in the use of African signs by Fani-Kayode and Hirst. Pollard, Duckworth, Mumtaz Karimjee and others use photography to speak about what it means to be a lesbian of colour, living on the cusp of racism and homophobia (Boffin and Fraser 1991, Karimjee 1991, Sulter 1990).

Many photographers have responded to the repression of lesbian sexuality by producing specifically sexual images. In doing so, they wrestle with the problem that pseudo-lesbian imagery is the staple of heterosexual male pornography, and that there are important issues of privacy, control and exploitation implicit in photographing the nude and/or sexualised female body. There is also often an unease with the sexual objectification of lesbian bodies, which too often appears to mimic the commodification of women's bodies within patriarchal images and texts. This unease can lead, ironically, to the denial of lesbian desire. For example Kate Millet, in her introduction to Cynthia MacAdams' book of nudes *Rising Goddess* (MacAdams 1983), says nothing about the possibility of lesbian desire being aroused by MacAdams' photographs, casting them rather as sexless images of one-ness with Nature and isolation from civilisation, despite the fact that MacAdam's camera dwells on her friends' bodies with a clear eroticism and that several of the photographs depict entwined lesbian couples!

More and more lesbian photographers are choosing to make specifically sexual lesbian work. Jill Posener, familiar as the anthologist of feminist graffiti, has begun contributing erotic photographs to lesbian sex magazine *On Our Backs*. Posener protested against Section 28 by photographing lesbians in sexual poses at famous London tourist attractions: a basque and suspender-clad dyke in fake fur coat lounges on the steps of the Albert Memorial, then changes into a leather jacket and joins her leather-clad girlfriend in erotic dalliance on Westminster Bridge, in the very shadow of the Houses of Parliament which would eradicate such acts.

A LESBIAN EROTIC GAZE?

Explicit photographs of lesbians as sexual agents may in and of themselves constitute acts of resistance against heteropatriarchal hegemony. Yet most lesbian erotic photography recycles a fairly familiar heterosexual semiotics. Sexual desire and agency have so long been constructed as masculine, sexual desireability has so long been coded on to/by means of the fetishised youthful female body, that a photograph which intends to say 'sex' has a hard time finding a new language to say it in. Lesbian photographers of the erotic for the most part rely heavily on a pre-existing economy of signs (as does gay male porn). Leather, garter belts, dildos, basques, fish-net stockings, spike-heeled shoes, black lace underwear, filmy, see-through material, tatoos, studs, chains and the paraphernalia of SM are all traditional signifiers of the hetero-erotic, and all are present in Della Grace's book *Love Bites* (Grace 1991). There is a certain amount of semiotic gender-fuck going on – a tutu teamed with a customised leather jacket, chains with net skirts, fish-net stockings with nine-hole Docs – but such sartorial trangressive-ness owes more to Punk than to lesbian-ness and makes for a peculiarly reactionary 'radicalism'. In the light of Madonna's *Sex*, the limited vocabulary of most lesbian erotic photography is clear.

It is a lot to ask of a photographer that she invent a new semiotics of sex, but many lesbian photographers are trying to do just that. Tee Corinne, using solarisation, reversed negatives and negative printing, has developed a technique for representing lesbian sexuality explicitly while refusing the pornographic vernacular (Boffin and Fraser 1991: 223–8). Some of Della Grace's later work dispenses with the hackneyed fetishism of *Love Bites*, photographing bald women, naked or partly so, in such a way as to downplay or erase entirely signifiers of gender. Works such as 'Triad' or 'Pussy-licking sodomite' (see *New Formations* 19: 125–30) do seem to offer the beginnings of a radically new way of photographing sexual lesbian-ness.

There are also the beginnings of a radically different contextual-isation of erotic imagery. In 1991, Kiss and Tell[7] published a postcard book, *Drawing the Line*, of their Canadian touring exhibition. The exhibition consisted of photographs of two members of Kiss and Tell in a variety of sexualised poses. Markers were provided and women invited to write comments on to the gallery walls, men into a book. The postcard book contains an invitation to readers to send in their comments on a pre-addressed card, and each photograph in the book carries a selection of the comments it engendered during the exhibition tour. The photographs thus become, in an innovative way, part of an interactive dialogue: 'We chose the postcard format as the best way to extend the interactive nature of the show' (Kiss and Tell 1991). In the face of often doctrinaire feminist attacks on lesbian sexual imagery (most feminist bookshops in Britain refuse to carry the lesbian sex magazine *Quim*, which publishes photographs by Laurence Jaugey-Paget, Della Grace and others), such openness is both courageous and necessary. Given the volatile nature of the erotic as a site for contestation around power, privilege, visibility and ethics, lesbian photography will long continue to be a fecund arena for cultural and political debate!

OUT ON SCREEN – LESBIANS AND FILM

There is no shortage of queer or feminist commentary on film, a situation which undoubtedly reflects the dominance of film studies within the academy in recent years. There is already a body of lesbian and gay film theory, criticism and commentary, with a growing list of publications (Bad Object-Choices 1991, Dyer 1990, Russo 1981), a few of which are specifically about lesbians in film (Weiss 1992, Wilton 1995). Thus, although lesbian-ness is still a marginal presence within film theory, there is more written on lesbians and film than on any other medium except literature. My focus here will be on the position of 'lesbian' in film theory debates.

The relative wealth of work on lesbian-ness in film is largely due to the nature of contemporary film theory, predicated as it is upon a psychoanalytic paradigm structured around heterobinarism. Within this paradigm the act of viewing film is understood as scopophilic – as a form of voyeurism, obtaining pleasure (which is understood to be sexual in kind) from the act of looking (Lapsley and Westlake 1988). Mainstream feminist and feminist-influenced film theory has developed an understanding of the cinematic apparatus as an intrinsically masculinist set of signifying practices, directing a (hetero)sexualised gaze at the female body and of cinema spectatorship as positioning the spectator as male within a heterosexual economy of desire and visual pleasure (Roof 1991). The cycle of spectatorship, the text/reader circuit, is reduced not only to a trading between men of looks-at-women, but also to a form of heterosexual activity. Castration anxiety is another psychoanalytic trope volubly present within film theory, presenting women as that-which-lacks-a-penis, or perceiving fetishism – a displacement activity to assuage castration fears – as associated with or embodied in the female object of the cinematic gaze (Stam *et al.* 1992). So not only heterosexuality but also *heterosexual masculinity* is seen as the subject of film: film becomes phallocentricity enacted/encoded. Women's presence on screen is no more than the making visible of a set of negotiations and affirmations of masculinity, as is her spectatorship of film.

Joan Riviere's notion of *masquerade* has been used by some film theorists to describe the positioning of women *vis-à-vis* film. By this analysis, femininity itself is no more than one way of being in respect of masculinity: 'to be a woman is to dissimulate a fundamental masculinity, femininity is that dissimulation' (Heath 1986 in Stam *et al.* 1992).

Clearly, this paradigm makes no space for 'lesbian'; whether as gazing subject or object of the gaze, 'she' must be merely male, merely female, her desire a mimesis of phallic potency, her desired body easily co-opted as properly feminine fetish. Either way, she is no more than a reminder/remainder of castration. Going beyond simple lesbian invisibility, lesbian spectacle/lesbian specularity are oxymoronic within this phallic project. In this, of course, 'lesbian' shares her impossibility with 'woman'. For, as Judith Roof notes:

> This has been the tendency in feminist film theory; to see representations of the female as inevitably bound up in an apparatus that operates primarily in a phallocentric field of sexual difference and which because of this, inevitably reproduces a phallocentric, and hence not female vision.
>
> (Roof 1991: 76)

Where may lesbians 'go', either in theorising or in producing film, if the filmic is intrinsically masculine? If, as Mulvey suggests, narrative film is constructed on 'the never fully-repressed bed-rock of feminine neurosis' (Mulvey 1989: 31), how may we achieve a feminist (let alone a lesbian) transformation of film? Mulvey insists that 'the female spectator . . . temporarily accepts "masculinization" in memory of her "active" phase . . . [her] phantasy of masculinization [is] at cross purposes with itself, restless in its transvestite clothes' (ibid.: 37). Accepting this, effectively renders impotent – because already masculinised – any attempt at gynocentric cinema. As Roof recognises:

> Theoretically, inscribing the cinematic apparatus as masculine makes dubious any possibility of representing a female perspective at all unless, as it might be argued, it is impossible to represent anything specifically female beyond a kind of textual practice consisting of a meditation on the nature of representation itself.
>
> (Roof 1991: 77)

She goes on to describe the two kinds of film-making which have developed in response to Mulvey's theoretical position, one which denies the scophophilic pleasure in looking and the other a 'completely analytical, metacritical practice' (ibid.). There has been, certainly in lesbian film-making, a third response; working explicitly with notions of lesbian looking and a lesbian gaze, and attempting to establish a radically different scopophilic dynamic – Sheila McLaughlin's *She Must Be Seeing Things* springs to mind here. But commentators disagree as to whether or not a lesbian cinematic gaze is possible, whether it disrupts or merely reinforces the hegemony of phallocentrism.

LESBIANS BUSY GAZING: ARE WE JUST BEING MEN AGAIN?

Ironically, it is within the excesses of phallocentrism that we may locate the possibility of a dykely rupture of this over-determined Freudianism. The heterosexual strai(gh)tjacket of psychoanalytic theory locates women's pleasure as *male-generated* in the circle of (heterosexual) spectatorship of pornographic film:

> Woman is given that orgasm and hence that phallus by men. . . . The male's phallus is the condition for female sexual pleasure . . . female sexual pleasure is the result ultimately of the gift of the phallus from members of the audience.
>
> (Ellis 1980, in Pajaczkowska 1992: 192)

Because he is writing about pornography, Ellis describes less euphemistically than most the heterosexual contract which is generally thought to structure film. That is, woman's pleasure lies in her (masochistic) awareness of her sexualised self as that-which-excites phallic sexuality – a kind of drawing down of male masturbatory potency. And it is in the relentless biological naivety of this metaphor that phallocentrism may be undone. For although the lesbian gaze may be re-coded as masculine, lesbian sexual pleasure resists reduction to the gift of a phallus by men.

Some commentators reject the suggestion that a lesbian presence in film may be disobedient, arguing that a lesbian gaze is always already incorporated into the dominant, heterosexual signifying economy and that hence it cannot escape reproducing the hegemony of phallocentric sexual/textual relations.

> 'Lesbian' viewing pleasure . . . is constructed around a set of over-determined relations between gender and sexuality; it does not exist outside of, but in complex relation to the 'deployment of sexuality' dominating contemporary discourse. 'Lesbian' appropriation of the 'gaze' comes only at the price of aquiescence to a system of sexual (gender and erotic) regularization that reproduces dominant taxonomies of sexual (gender and erotic) difference.
>
> (Traub 1991: 308)

If the gaze is accepted as intrinsically masculine, and the cinematic apparatus as both regulated by and reproducing the taxonomic binaries of the heteropatriarchal sex/gender system, then this is undoubtedly (and by definition) so. If the cultural arena is always already structured along a polarity of gender, 'lesbian' as a position or positions along the axis of that polarity inevitably acquiesces to its hegemony. However, if we refuse this (patriarchal) positioning of 'lesbian', taking rather a position eccentric to the male/female axis – 'outside the heterosexual social contract', as Teresa de Laurietis puts it (in Roof 1991: 51) – a more complex, perhaps fractal, model of the multiple intersections of gender/desire/acts/identities becomes possible.

Once we accept the possibility that 'desire itself is not heterosexually monolithic' (Roof 1991), the lesbian position becomes something quite different:

> This is what the lesbian configuration reveals. There is more to sexuality and sexual difference than the mere fact of gender; desire and sexual orientation already destabilize any binary system and with it any necessary hegemony of the heterosexually premised machine.
>
> (Roof 1991: 50)

Within this model a kind of chaos geometry of desire emerges, a complexity whose logic is not amenable to the limited apperceptions of binarism. Freeing film and film theory from the Freudian straitjacket of castration-fetish dialectics also reveals a quite different 'film':

> If mastery and disavowal of lack are not necessarily the prime movers of cinema, if we unmoor theories of the cinematic apparatus from their fixation on sexual difference, their privileging of mastery and their fixation on sexual castration, we might see how the apparatus is both more problematically and more intricately self-contradictory.
>
> (ibid.: 51)

Although Roof still writes in Freudian terms, her theory of viewing pleasure takes account of 'the uncontrollably multiple identifications created by the interference of unstable sexual identities' (ibid.: 51–2). Here 'lesbian' occupies a uniquely powerful position, precisely because the lesbian desiring gaze simultaneously *of* and *at* a woman contradicts utterly the heterosexual master narrative. Traub suggests:

> In the context of theorizing a gaze unbound by rigid gender polarities, the figure of the 'lesbian' is, it seems to me, a privileged site of inquiry. As both subject and object of desire, she embodies the potential desiring modality of all viewing subjects, her body displacing the binary economy enforced by heterosexual ideology.
>
> (Traub 1991: 311)

Traub does not suggest that this privileged 'lesbian' is able to dispense with the heterosexual binary altogether, 'the "lesbian" *subverts* but cannot *overturn* the hegemony of binary codes'. This, for Traub, is because 'lesbian' is still 'constrained by the structural asymmetries of gender'.

It is clearly not possible here to resolve the question of whether a lesbian gaze is a catalyst for the transformation of heterosexual binarism in film/film theory or whether it is merely a disobedient presence within that still hegemonic binary. I would like to finish this brief lesbian foray into the opacities of film theory with an interesting comment from Teresa de Lauretis, which suggests to me that the position of 'lesbian' in film theory has yet to be adequately understood:

> [T]he notion of female sexuality as fluid, diffuse, polymorphously perverse, or mobile and unbounded, is applicable to lesbian sexuality only if the above qualifiers are not, as they usually are, taken to be equivalent to bisexual. For it seems to me that this notion of female bisexuality, with its emphasis on androgyny – or a blurring of the boundaries between male-sexed and female-sexed bodies, or of the boundaries of gender that, wishful theorizing notwithstanding, do stick to the sexed body in one way or another – is itself a fantasy. And not a very engaging fantasy for lesbians.
>
> (de Lauretis 1991: 237–8)

This suggestion – that a refusal of androgyny is as important to lesbian-ness as the refusal of masculine desire – opens up a multitude of new questions concerning the specificity of lesbian desire and the lesbian gaze, and the precise nature of its absolute distinction from heterosexual female sexuality. Lesbian film theory is clearly on the edge of some exciting developments.

PERFORMING IDENTITIES: MUSIC AND LESBIAN CULTURE

Music, dance and theatre all stand in somewhat peculiar relation to lesbian-ness. All are stereotypically identified with gay men – the opera queen, the disco diva, the ballet dancer and the actor are all staples both of camp celebration and of homophobic rhetoric. Music is apparently an important ingredient of lesbian social life, yet it is profoundly difficult to excavate either lesbian producers and performers or a lesbian theoretical position on music. There is no lesbian equivalent of Michael Clark, John Gielgud or Wayne Sleep, and although there are lesbian plays and theatre groups they lack the cultural visibility of *Bent* or *Torch Song Trilogy* (though see Rapi 1990 and 1991, Melville n.d.). A queer scholarship of the performing arts is developing (see de Jongh 1992), and there are certainly important avenues of enquiry around lesbian theatre and dance, but since there is somewhat less of a silence concerning music than the others, and since music is so significant in lesbian social-ising, it is with music that this section mostly engages. Which is not to suggest that lesbian/gay musicology is a thriving field: the first book on the subject (Brett *et al.* 1995) is a somewhat late arrival on the queer academic scene, whilst dedicated queer musicologist Jay McClaren, beavering away in Amsterdam on his *Encyclopaedia of Gay and Lesbian Recordings* has been 'surprised at the resistance to my concept' among publishers and has been forced to distribute the *Encyclopaedia* privately, in the form of a limited edition chap book (McClaren 1992).

Elite or 'classical' music does not play the same part in lesbian life as it does in gay men's, something which reflects the relative privilege of gay men in a patriarchal culture. Not only is their earning power greater than that of lesbians, but the overwhelming majority of cultural producers, interpreters, performers and consumers are men. Simple statistics would suggest that many of these men would be gay; in addition, the ascribed effeminacy of the 'arts', together with a permitted bohemianism, a privileged moral laxity and the traditional exclusion of women, have long made theatres and concert halls in the West sanctuaries for gay men (Garrard 1976, McClary 1991).

There are, as usual, two critical strands of interest to lesbians wishing to engage with 'classical' music, the queer and the feminist. Neither makes much theoretical space for 'lesbian'. It is left to lesbian studies to engage with the intersection of gender, sexuality and music which a lesbian prespective mandates.

The historical absolute exclusion of women from participation in Western music is clearly inextricable from the wider social control of women. As Jane Bowers tells us:

> On 4 May 1686 Pope Innocent XI issued an edict which declared that 'music is completely injurious to the modesty that is proper for the female sex, because they become distracted from the matters and occupations most proper for them.' Therefore, 'no unmarried woman, married woman or widow of any rank, status, condition, even those who for reasons of education or anything else are living in convents or conservatories, under any pretext, even to learn music in order to practise it in those convents, may learn to sing from men . . . and to play any sort of musical instrument'.
>
> (Bowers 1986: 139–40)

The fluctuating conception of music as either proper or improper for women gives rise to and is itself shaped by an unstable gendering of music itself, a gendering that reflects the kaleidoscopic anxieties which group and regroup around masculinity and the abject feminine in a series of historical crises. As McClary notes, 'some women composers of so-called serious or experimental music are discovering many of the forms and conventional procedures of presumably value-free music are saturated with hidden patriarchal narratives, images, agendas' (McClary 1991: 154). While it is almost impossible to locate lesbian-ness in the history of this co-option,[8] it is important to insert 'lesbian' into theories of music as gendered, in order to pre-empt the reification of music-as-heterosexual. This is perhaps especially important in opera which one feminist critic has characterised as 'bourgeois, nationalist, femicidal, expensive' (Hasted 1989). While recognising the political limitations of opera, it may be possible to carve out an operatic space – however illicit – for lesbian scavenging:

> In a world where women are too often silenced, a soprano voice hitting the back wall of a huge, silent auditorium in a wave of pure sound, conveying rage, joy, pain, grief or desire, can send shivers down my spine.
>
> (Hasted 1989: 37)

To refuse to see the significance of this privileged and exclusive space for women making a noise is to fail to grasp both a patriarchal strategy (the bird in the gilded cage?) and a possible site of female strength.

Feminist music theory is developing exciting insights into the ways in which gender is mapped on to musical form – tonality, modality, rhythm – and hence into possibilities for a musical form resistant to masculine interpretation (see McClary 1991), but I am not aware that any of this work incorporates a lesbian focus, nor of any theoretical explorations of the work of lesbian composers. This work remains to be done. Queer music theory, interdisciplinary in its approach, offers some equally useful interpretations. Wayne Koestenbaum sees parallels between the act of singing and the act of being homosexual:

> [T]he homosexual body, whether silent or vocal, occupies a crossroads where anatomies and institutions collide. Like voice, homosexuality appears to be taking place inside a body, when really it occurs in a sort of outerspace (call it 'discourse') where interiorities converge; the vocal body and the homosexual body each appear to be a membraned box of urges, when actually each is a looseleaf rulebook, a ledger of inherited prohibitions.
>
> (Koestenbaum 1991: 207)

The 'ledger of inherited prohibitions', so graphically described by Koestenbaum, is different for lesbians and gay men. Importantly, the prohibitions adhere to regulatory axes such as class and race as well as to gender and sexuality. Yet his insistence on the physicality of singing is an important one and points to a long-overdue reinscription of the body into theories of sexuality.

As far as formal music theory is concerned, lesbian scholarship is in its infancy. Queer is just beginning to intervene in musicology, and feminist music theory is still relatively unfamiliar within women's studies. It remains for lesbian studies to initiate a specifically lesbian musicology.

THE SINGER OR THE SONG? DYKES IN POPULAR MUSIC

Popular music appears to saturate lesbian social life. From the establishment of the US women's music industry, with its independent production and distribution apparatus (Shapiro 1978) to the kd lang phenomenon of butch chic, popular music has woven an affirmative strand against the homophobia of the mainstream. In some sense, pop culture has developed of late a self-consciously anti-homophobic agenda, with publications like *The Face* and cultural activism such as Pop Against Homophobia (PAH) (Daniel and Brill 1991)[9] attempting to eradicate homophobia by labelling it uncool and untrendy, much as earlier campaigns challenged racism. Anti-homophobic pop-cultural activism generally reflects a more sophisticated awareness of class and race than the more academic arena of Cultural Studies.

Lesbian interests have been particularly well served within pop music.[10] Since the early 1970s, the independent women's music industry, comprising businesses such as Wise Women's Enterprises Inc., Olivia Records, Women's Revolutions Per Minute, Ladyslipper and Redwood Records, has recorded and distributed women's music, and women's music festivals are highspots of the US lesbian calendar. Much of this music is by, for and about lesbians, and a significant part of the labour force within this alternative industry is lesbian (Shapiro 1978). Singers such as Holly Near, Alix Dobkin, Chris Williamson and Meg Christian should be seen as belonging to the wider lesbian-feminist activism of the 1970s, one of a kind with lesbian-feminist publishing houses and other lesbian-run small businesses. The lesbian music industry was part of a general separatist strategy.

This early separatism is worlds away from kd lang's insouciant disregard for gender. Claiming that she doesn't care whether men or women are attracted to her, lang playfully admits to 'a little bit of penis envy. They're ridiculous, but they're cool' (Bennetts 1993: 51). Her butch cool owes more to the gender-fuck of Boy George, Prince or Annie Lennox than to lesbian feminism. It is unclear whether her success indicates the fragility of the confidence of heteropatriarchal values. In commenting that 'Nashville couldn't cope [with lang undercutting] all the old stereotypes of femininity, gender, and sexual preference' (ibid.: 50), the *Vanity Fair* article is demonstrating that the magazine and its readers *can* cope. 'Look', the article is saying, 'lesbians aren't scary at all'.

The 1970s tradition of independent music-making goes on, with local lesbian bands – such as The Friggin' Little Bits from Northern England – coming together and disbanding soon after. Groups often record songs on audio cassette for distribution in women's bookshops and at concerts. Such cassettes pass, by a process of re-recording on personal tape decks, throughout sub-groups of the lesbian community, gradually losing sound quality as they go. In the USA, where the relative size of the lesbian population supports a music industry which is more of a free market, lesbian recording artists such as Ferron or Phranc are available on vinyl or even CD, and cross the Atlantic to become cherished lesbian cult figures. Such singers, relatively unknown in mainstream pop circles, take on the status of in-group secret in lesbian communities. However, many young lesbians apparently prefer straight disco music (Bradby 1993) to avowedly and self-consciously lesbian music, while Jay McClaren notes that 'most gay men and lesbians do not choose to buy gay records. They are more likely to buy a book with gay content or watch a TV programme with gay references, but they happily buy "straight" music' (McClaren 1992: Introduction).

NEVER MIND THE MUSIC, FEEL THE STYLE

As musicologist Susan McClary has noted, it is seldom the actual *music* of pop performers which is commented on in cultural criticism. Rather, it is the image, the style, the presentation (McClary 1991). Perhaps this is why the heterosexual Madonna receives so much more queer attention than lesbian singers such as Bessie Smith, Ma Rainey or Ferron. Thus, for example, although McClary's own analysis of Madonna's music shows the Material Girl to be 'an expert in the arena of musical signifi-cation' and one who is 'engaged in rewriting some very fundamental levels of Western thought' (McClary 1991: 160–1) – all of which is interesting, but none of which is readily accessible to the superficial analysis of queer – it is Madonna's image, presented in her videos, films and (especially) her photobook *Sex* (Madonna 1992), which have engaged queer critics (see Frank and Smith 1993, Schwichtenberg 1993). Interestingly, gay writer Simon Frith condemns Madonna as a musician for exactly those attributes which McClary identifies as ground-breaking – her refusal to be controlled musically within and by the production conventions of pop.

This focus on image to the exclusion of the music itself is dominant in the lesbian reponse to performers. We ignore the possibility that Madonna is a 'woman musician who can create images of desire without the demand within the discourse itself that she be destroyed' (McClary 1991), and debate instead her presentation of her body and sexuality (Frank and Smith 1993). We remain silent about kd lang's voice and concentrate on how she 'bends gender cliches' (Bennetts 1993), and when Phranc is interviewed for a lesbian magazine she is asked one question about her music and sixteen about such burning issues as how good she is in bed, whether Martina and kd really *are* an item, or whether she is butch (Delores 1993).

The apparent centrality of lesbian music to lesbian culture is illusory. Music is as important to lesbians (and to gay men) as to any other sub-cultural group. That is to say, young urban dykes whose social lives revolve around clubs, older professional lesbians whose social lives revolve around wining and dining, or lesbians of colour whose lives are as structured by racism as by homophobia, all have very different relationships to music. The question for lesbian studies about popular music has been framed by Barbara Bradby: '*Why and how the question of authorship matters in the lives of those who live the particular culture*' (Bradby 1993: 151, emphasis in original). It may well be that taste in music is as little amenable to political conviction as sexual desire, a point recognised by Tom Robinson, of Glad to be Gay fame: 'I've found the established gay scene to be more or less indifferent to my music. Basically, you follow your taste in music rather than the sexual preference of the performer' (Robinson 1989: 278). He also recognises that, ironically, mainstream performers with what he calls a 'watered down' gay message, may offer more to young gay listeners than openly gay performers:

> David Bowie waters the message down and gets from one end of the earth to the other. When Bowie came up with *Hunky Dory* fifteen years ago, I knew what he was talking about and it affected my life in

an enormous way. Had that message been stronger, and not broadcast on the radio, I'd never have heard it.

(ibid.: 279)

This opens up important questions about access to the broadcast media and about the relative significance of openly gay performers whose music is popular in its own right and with a mainstream audience. The queer presence on broadcast media is increasing, with gay cable channels in the USA and regular lesbian and gay series on Channel 4 in Britain. Even the BBC has opened out of late, with several one-off lesbian and gay programmes on television and radio and, at the time of writing, a regular lesbian and gay programme slot on Radio 1, its mass audience pop station.

This moving into the mainstream does not indicate an unproblematic increase in the visibility of lesbians. Heterosexism is a peculiarly resilient phenomenon, characterised by a stubborn ability to re-code to its own ends. Even the 'reading' of an obviously gay performer like Julian Clary may be informed by homophobia in complex and subtle ways: some of my students refuse to accept that Clary is gay, preferring to believe that he is 'just acting'. Given that Clary is publicly unambiguous about his sexuality this reascription of his heterosexuality represents a reading against the grain quite as muscular as that of any lesbian attempting to fit Madonna into a dyke-shaped hole!

CONCLUSION

Music, art and film offer many questions for Lesbian Studies: questions about authorship, the gendering of the medium and of the apparatus of representation, the sexual and erotic politics of music-making or mark-making, the permeable boundary between the mainstream and the 'oppositional', co-option, disobedient readings and the historical presence of lesbians in the visual and performing arts. Cultural studies is an important site of lesbian intervention, while lesbian studies, with its familiarity with scavenging, re-inscription, reading against the grain and re-coding, has a specifically disobedient astringency to offer the discipline.

NOTES

1 Admittedly, this is an assumption of mine . . . but the object in question is considerably longer than 12 inches, which outdoes anything I have had the pleasure of subjecting to the lesbian gaze, even in gay men's porn.

2 Although Nochlin does later in her paper suggest that living with a 'sympathetic' woman friend who 'did not demand the same sacrifice of genuine
   commitment to her profession which marriage would have entailed' was
   useful in enabling Bonheur to follow her art, she sees it as a contraceptive
   strategy: 'The advantages of such an arrangement for women who wished
   to avoid the distraction of children in the days before reliable contraception
   are obvious' (Nochlin 1989: 173). Simple, really. I don't know why nobody
   has thought of it before – now we have effective contraception we don't
   need to be lesbians.
3 To identify the man's behaviour rather than the woman's love for him as the
   source of pain may not seem to be a specifically lesbian insight, but the
   plethora of books aimed at 'women who love too much', together with other
   feminist analyses in a psychoanalytic paradigm (for example, Orbach and
   Eichenbaum 1983), indicate a growing tendency to pathologise women's
   love for men within the context of heterosexuality.
4 For information about this British group write to P.O. Box 2DL, London
   W1A 2DL, UK.
5 Perhaps I should declare a bias here, since I am a lesbian cartoonist myself.
   Not that this clouds my judgement – cartooning is self-evidently a truly
   wonderful art!
6 Of course, there is a book or two to be written about why there is no lesbian
   equivalent of Tom of Finland – not to mention a lesbian-feminist critique of
   his work, which has much to say about constructions of masculinity and
   contains some surprising reworking of gender codes.
7 A collaboration between Susan Stewart, photographer, and Persimmon
   Blackridge and Lizard Jones.
8 Although I have a personal suspicion about Hildegard von Bingen
   (1098–1179), a visionary, poet, mystic, naturalist, healer, theologian and
   musician, who established three covents and wrote music which I can only
   describe as saturated with female spirituality. Her works are available in
   modern recordings, and well worth a lesbian ear. For a feminist biography,
   see Flanagan (1989).
9 Pop Against Homophobia is a small-scale organisation which produces
   posters, postcards and T-shirts depicting lesbian and gay-positive images. It
   describes itself as a 'youth culture advertising campaign' and says 'PAH
   advertising campaigns are launched throughout the world and feature images of affectionate same-sex couples, images which are usually censored
   by the media and advertising companies' (from back of PAH postcard,
   1992). The campaign is probably unique in that it makes overt use of the
   capitalist institution, one of its aims being to 'reveal the positive use of
   same-sex relationship lifestyles to marketing and advertising companies in
   their promotions'. PAH may be contacted at: 3rd Floor, 104–8 Bolsover
   Street, London W1P 7HF.
10 I am using 'pop' music in the generalist way 'classical' music is often used.
   In what follows, 'pop' encompasses funk, rock, heavy metal, folk, blues,
   jazz, rap, country, etc., as well as what might be called 'real pop' (as in,
   'Madonna is a pop singer, not a rock singer').

Chapter 8

The social lesbian

For us, love is not the same; sex is not the same; parenting is not the same; work is not the same; safety is not the same; respect is not the same; trust is not the same. Only death might, perhaps, be the same.
(Namjoshi and Hanscombe 1986)

LESBIANS AND SOCIOLOGY

There has been comparatively little lesbian intervention in sociology. Yet sociology has much to offer as a framework for describing and understanding the social position of lesbians. Why, then, this tradition of non-involvement?

Although it has traditionally had a critique of socio-economic inequality, sociology, as part of the enlightenment rationlist project, developed in the interests of an elite which identified itself as the norm. Sociological discourse and praxis have been unexaminedly racist, sexist and heterosexist. The nature of sociology as a study of human groups and societies imposed an additional inequity. In the hierarchy of the research process the researcher's 'expert' status made him/her superior to the object of study (the criminal, the teenager, the prostitute, the homosexual), a polarisation which functioned both to construct and reinforce the 'otherness' of the object studied and to naturalise its own operation. It is only comparatively recently, with the rise of an identity politics originating with the Black civil rights movement and the so-called second wave of the women's movement, that the marginalised and objectified have been asserting their subjecthood and troubling the boundaries between researcher and researched. For example, Nickie Charles outlines the changes that have taken place in sociology in reponse to feminist intervention:

It has been suggested that the relationship between feminism and the social sciences can be divided into four phases. The first is the pre-feminist era when women were almost totally neglected as objects of study; the second is marked by the emergence of a critique of this neglect; in the third stage research is undertaken on women in order to 'add them on' to existing studies; and the fourth consists of a full theoretical integration of gender into the discipline.

(Charles 1993: 2)

I would suggest an additional, more political achievement: feminism has revealed the complicity of putatively neutral social scientific discourse in the tautological reification of 'woman' and has shown that this operates in the interests of male supremacy (Birke 1992, Bleier 1991, Thiele 1992). Faraday (1981) suggests that this is also true of research into lesbians. Feminist social scientists have developed a specifically feminist research praxis, characterised by reflexivity and an awareness of the power dynamic inherent in the research process (Gross 1992, Kelly *et al.* 1992, Mies 1983, Oakley 1980, Stanley 1992).

It is against this general insistence that social scientific discourse is a site of struggle over meanings (and, moreover, of those meanings as constitutive and expressive of relations of *power*) that the emergence of lesbian sociology must be seen. Lesbian scholars have suggested ways in which the deployment of the lesbian-as-stigmatised-other functions within the social institution of gender to oppress all women (Faraday 1981, Radicalesbians 1970, Wittig 1981) while recognising (as heterosexual feminists tend not to do) the specifics of the social position of lesbians. Much of this commentary (though by no means all) has taken place outwith the academy, or at least outwith the epistemological structures of mainstream sociology. Rather it has been located within 'feminist theory' and seen as a multi-disciplinary (or supra-disciplinary) project.

Disobedience to the doctrines and regulations of the male academy is characteristic of feminist scholarship, and an active engagement with questions of disciplinary boundaries which foregrounds the motivation and consequences of their construction is part and parcel of the feminist critique of the academy. This political stance certainly contributes to the current situation whereby, although lesbian feminist theory often engages with issues which fall within the field of the social sciences, social scientific enterprise of a more formal nature remains relatively empty of lesbian participation.

Sociology has recently begun to engage in exciting new ways with the question of sexuality. The prestigious British Sociological Association annual conference in 1994 took 'Sexualities in Social Context' as its theme, and it is within sociology that the anti-essentialist model of sexual identity has been developed. However, the social sciences are perceived by many lesbians as intrinsically homophobic and, indeed, stigma continues to confront the researcher into lesbian and gay sociology. As Ken Plummer points out in the first published British collection to deal with the sociology of homosexuality:

> Since homosexuality in this culture remains largely 'taboo' and subject to hostility and attack, it is not surprising that those who elect to conduct research into this area will also be subject to such condemnation. . . . Anybody embarking upon such research – gay or not – should thus give serious consideration to being 'dis-creditable' or 'discredited'.
>
> (Plummer 1981b: 226–7)

The stigma assigned to same-sex affectional/erotic behaviour and the concomitant professional risk to individuals studying such behaviour has policed the academy as effectively as any other arena of social life, severely limiting research activity in this area as it limits sexual activity in the private sphere. Plummer's more recent work suggests that there has been little improvement:

> Our enemies are everywhere – it is hard to get funding, people would like to stop us doing our work, we may not get tenure, people look with suspicion on lesbian and gay causes, there is employment discrimination, and so on.
>
> (Plummer 1992: 12)

The beleaguered status of queer scholarship clearly makes developing a lesbian sociology extremely difficult. Add to this the disadvantaged position of women within the academy, and perhaps it becomes clear why so few lesbian researchers ventured into the field for so long. There are gender-related constraints for the lesbian sociologist which are additional to the problems experienced by gay men. Women have traditionally been excluded from social science research both as object and subject (Abbott and Wallace 1990), and educational institutions have systematically directed girls and young women away from the sciences and towards the arts and humanities (Kelly 1987, Orr 1985, Scott 1980). Thus, while it is unusual to find gay men researching gay issues in the social sciences, a lesbian in the field is of mythological rarity – a veritable unicorn among scholars (Faraday 1981).

This depressing picture is currently undergoing dramatic change. Primarily in the United States but also in the European mainland and in Britain, the academy has witnessed a growing queer momentum in the social sciences. In this chapter I want to sketch a brief outline of this shift and to assess the workings of what may be increasingly recognised as a dynamic interface between the lesbian and the social.

A SOCIOLOGY OF LESBIANISM – SOME QUEERIES

Sociology is 'the study of human social life, groups and societies' (Giddens 1989: 7). As such, it has the potential to be a radical and liberatory project (and has certainly acquired a somewhat suspect status as 'political' in the eyes of politicians and the press). Its scope, as Giddens comments, 'is extremely wide, ranging from the analysis of passing encounters between individuals in the street up to the investigation of global social processes' (ibid.: 8). Some developments in sociological theory – symbolic interactionism for example – are particularly useful to lesbians. Interactionism studies meaning-making as a social activity, something of great interest to anyone concerned with the competing meanings of sexuality and gender.

Sociology has not yet, however, exploited its radical potential to the full. In her important essay 'Liberating lesbian research' Annabel Faraday assesses the inadequacy of the social sciences in dealing with lesbians. She identifies four major failings:

- the assumption that a lesbian is no more than a 'female homosexual' and that anything said about gay men will unproblematically apply to her with few, if any, reservations.
- the adoption of a male-defined model of sexuality as referent and paradigm.
- the chronic androcentrism of academic discourse which relegates all women, lesbians included, to the status of footnote.
- the 'invisibility' of lesbians to scrutiny is attributed to their unwillingness (relative to gay men) to enter the public sphere, socially or for sexual activity, rather than to the heteropatriarchal power structures which confine and restrict the activity of *all* women.

(Faraday 1981)

In other words, an adequate epistemological matrix for lesbian research has to be developed from a specifically feminist perspective on sex and gender, which includes an imperative to recognise and deconstruct the 'otherness' of lesbians *as women* in the context of the study of homosexuality. It is perhaps ironic that Faraday's protest was ever necessary, given widespread awareness among queer academics that sociology (in common with all other academic disciplines) has not itself given up constructing the homosexual-as-other.

THE BAD OLD DAYS

Sociological inquiry into homosexuality is a recent phenomenon, spanning only forty or so years. The earliest studies which may loosely be termed 'sociological' are those of the sexologists, particularly Kinsey, and these tended to problematise the aetiology of same-sex desire, thus reinforcing the hegemonic status of heterosexuality. Slightly later mainstream sociological research became interested in questions of stigma and related issues of primary and secondary deviance. Typical of this trend was the heterosexual researcher examining homosexuality in parallel with prostitution, hooliganism, illegal drug use and criminality, from the perspective of what is now known as labelling theory.[1]

The entire arena of the sexual has long been seen as an inappropriate and suspect field for academic investigation (Masters and Johnson 1979). Added to this general opprobrium, the stigma and illegality of homosexuality made it a potentially contaminating field of study. Researchers took pains to stress their own heterosexuality (Humphreys 1970, Ponse 1978, Wolf 1979), often working such declarations into the conventions of academic discourse in a way that is both blatant and apparently subtle. Strategies include dedicating books to their spouses and children (often with the implication that it was only with the restorative presence of a normal family that they were able to venture safely into such queer territory), discussing the difficulties they faced as outsiders doing research into sub-cultural groups, or reflecting on the ethics of their exploitation (as privileged heterosexuals) of a vulnerable group.

The dangers are all too real: heterosexual researchers have been dissuaded from work in the field by threats to the custody of their children, to 'their tenure, promotion, reputation and personal safety' (Harbeck 1992). Clearly, with penalties of this nature visited on heterosexuals for even presuming to *study* homosexuality, the potential risks for scholars who were themselves lesbian or gay precluded their involvement in such work (Wolf 1979). Other considerations which prevented lesbians conducting scholarly research into their own communities included the belief that to do so would expose them to accusations of special pleading (Wolf 1979), or a rejection of the academic enterprise in toto as irredeemably masculinist (Lorde 1979, Radicalesbians 1970) and hence not only merely diversionary but actively collusive with women's oppression.

Heterosexual dominance in a precarious field resulted in the loss of lesbian/gay control over methodology, data collected and the uses to which it might be put. There were (and still are) important political and ethical dimensions to research done into (sometimes 'on behalf of') oppressed and marginalised groups. A good example here is Laud Humphreys' *The Tearoom Trade*, an early (1970) account of his participant observation research into casual male homosexual encounters in American public toilets. Humphreys' ethnographic methodology involved active deception, collaboration with the police and the adoption of a fake persona. He posed as an accomplice, a lookout, in order to enable him to spend long periods of time in public toilets observing clandestine (and illegal) sexual encounters, and followed up individual men for further questioning. 'By noting registration numbers of cars belonging to the participants, and with some help from the police, he was able to discover their addresses and interview the men subsequently, ostensibly for an innocuous survey unconnected with homosexuality' (Humphreys 1970: vii). Humphreys was aware of the ethical issues raised and declared his methodology justified in the light of his declared intention to use the information he gained to further scientific knowledge (ibid.: 172–3).

There can be no doubt that the data collected by Humphreys was significant on two counts: it cast doubt on the necessary coterminosity of homosexual acts and identities (the majority of men observed in the study were married and identified firmly as *heterosexual*), and it exposed the inaccuracy of the myth of the homosexual as predator on or recruiter of heterosexuals. Humphreys himself made use of his findings to call in no uncertain terms for a liberalisation of the laws criminalising male homosexual acts (ibid.: 163–6). Nevertheless, the men involved lacked any degree of knowledge of or control over the research process and its findings, and this remains problematic.

LIBERAL TOLERANCE AND RADICAL CHALLENGE: THE GROUND SHIFTS

In the USA in 1965, a popular account, *Lesbianism in America*, was published by a gay man, Donald Cory and was widely read (Wolf 1979). As a gay man, Cory's motivation was to encourage sympathy among the wider community for same-sex eroticism, something common to most (if not all) such accounts published outside the specialist market in the 1960s and 1970s. Certainly, the accounts of many of the early hetero-sexual writers on lesbianism were philanthropic and/or advocative in intent, motivated by a desire (couched in more or less academic language) to enable the non-lesbian world to *understand the lesbian*. Ponse is typical:

> In the pages that follow, I will attempt to take the reader through the process of comprehending the meanings of lesbian, moving from a common-sense point of view external to the lesbian world to an appreciation of the complexity of identity formation among women who love women.
>
> (Ponse 1978: 22)

This assimilationist account, aiming for (heterosexual) tolerance, was central to the homophile politics of the time and marked an important step in gay liberation. A contemporary reading notes the unproblematic assumption of a heterosexual audience, the positioning of non-lesbian as 'common-sense' and the refusal to consider that identity formation among women who love men may also contain 'complexity'. By such unexamined textual practice is 'otherness' constituted!

It would be incorrect to suggest that this set of attitudes is now defunct (although obsolete). Barrett, for example, writes in 1990 of her motivation to share with her fellow heterosexuals her recognition that, '(lesbians) were women just as "nice" as straight women who were forced to hide in double lives, unable to share their hopes, joys and disappointments because of hostility, prejudice and ignorance' (Barrett 1990: 16). Researchers such as Ponse and Barrett undoubtedly mean well, but the inadequacy and ultimately reactionary nature of their agenda is exposed by their bewilderment when faced with lesbian 'meanings'. Ponse, for example, is at first unable to understand why her own sexuality should be an issue of concern among her researchees: 'I was . . . discomfited by the focus on my identity on whether I was gay or not. I couldn't see why that mattered' (Ponse 1978: 15); and although, to give her her due, she does record the changes which took place in her understanding of this, she never quite gets the point.

However problematic heterosexual research into lesbianism may be, there is no justification for suggesting that it should not take place. The mountain of publications on the sociology of lesbians is not so massive that we can afford to close any avenues and, in any case, such texts offer ready material for those who seek to problematise heterosexism. There have been, too, heterosexual writers whose work has demonstrated admirable openness to lesbian meanings. Deborah Goleman Wolf, for example (1979), takes on with gusto the task of *describing* (rather than explaining) a US lesbian-feminist community, offering it as a model of good practice for those who wish to build cohesive and succesful small urban communities (and the implication is certainly that such an audience will include lesbians as well as non-lesbians) rather than interpreting it as an alien phenomenon to and for the benefit of the dominant group. It is Wolf's feminism which enables her to recognise and represent the political nature of the community she describes. However, within mainstream academic discourse, lesbianism continued until very recently to be constructed in terms which were collusive with the mechanics of lesbian oppression. Articles about homosexuality in general and lesbians in particular were most often to be found in such publications as the *Journal of Abnormal and Social Psychology* and the *British Journal of Psychiatry* or in books with names like *Sexual Deviance and Sexual Deviants* (Goode and Troiden 1974), or *The Problem of Homosexuality in Modern Society* (Ruitenback 1963).

This changed with the growth of civil rights movements. Black Power, 'second wave' feminism, the post-Stonewall lesbian and gay movement all came into being in a few extraordinary years. A new radicalism took root in the academy, challenging pedagogic practices and the academic curriculum. Students were sprayed with Mace and tear gas, beaten and shot. There was optimism that radical practitioners could challenge and transform the oppressive discourses of the social sciences.

FROM THE HORSE'S MOUTH: QUEER SOCIOLOGISTS

Probably the earliest attempt by lesbians to subject lesbian life to rudimentary social-scientific scrutiny was the 1959 survey conducted by the San Francisco branch of the first lesbian social/political group, the Daughters of Bilitis (DOB). The report was based on replies to a questionnaire sent to readers of the *Ladder*, the DOB newsletter, and was therefore limited to a self-selected sub-group within the embryonic lesbian sub-culture, but it was truly a ground-breaking enterprise and one which was not to be followed for a dozen or so years (Wolf 1979). In 1972 two books, Del Martin and Phyllis Lyon's *Lesbian/Woman* and Sidney Abbott and Barbara Love's *Sappho Was a Right-On Woman: A Liberated View of Lesbianism*, were published in the USA – although the original publisher refused to accept the final manuscript of Martin and Lyon's book because it did not conclude by rejecting lesbianism! These two books set the tone for what was to become a slowly increasing trickle of lesbian-authored accounts of lesbian lives in a heterosexist society. Such accounts were targeted at a lesbian audience and, therefore, many are informal and popular in character, rather than making any attempt at formal social-scientific analysis. Lesbian sociology rapidly developed a theoretical base, however, and by 1984 it was possible for Trudy Darty and Sandee Potter to publish *Women-Identified Women*, an edited collection of essays which ranged from literary criticism to accounts of lesbians in the labour market and which included many research-based sociological pieces.

Lesbian sociological writings were often constructed around auto-biographical accounts (for example, Vida 1978). This trend continued through the 1970s and 1980s right up to the present day (see, for example, Porter and Weeks 1991, National Lesbian and Gay Survey 1992). Although it is certainly possible to interpret, edit or re-write autobiographical accounts to fit a pre-existing theory, by and large such acounts enable a more diverse and complex set of meanings to be constructed from among their polyvocal narratives. As well as challenging the inequitable power relations between researcher and researched,[2] autobiography offers one important way to explore the differences and diversity which have been recognised as important issues for lesbians and for any attempt to forge a lesbian community.

Perhaps ironically, the collection of autobiographical accounts has gained (contested) credibility within the methodology of the formal social sciences, enabling social scientific accounts based on lesbian and gay autobiography to take a place in the academic canon. In Britain the Hall Carpenter Archives Lesbian Oral History Group (1991) and the National Lesbian and Gay Survey (1992) have both published collections of lesbian autobigraphy, while in the USA, the Gay and Lesbian Advocacy Research Project gives much weight to autobiographical accounts in its publication *Growing Up Gay in the South* (Sears 1991). Oral history and personal accounts also have developed into a valued and important trend in historical work and here, too, lesbian and gay scholarship has contibuted (Neild and Pearson 1992, Porter and Weeks 1991).

Moving beyond describing what it was like to live as a lesbian, lesbian-authored texts in the 1970s and early 1980s began to discuss heterosexism, the legal position of lesbians, the relationship between sex and gender, the development of theories of lesbianism in psychology/ sexology/biology, etc. and many other directly relevent issues (Abbott and Love 1972, Darty and Potter 1984, Klaich 1985), as professionally educated lesbians began to direct their formal, scholarly gaze towards lesbian-ness. While the project of informing lesbians about other lesbian lives continues, there has been an increasing involvement of lesbian academics in foregrounding lesbianism as a topic for scholarly debate and study within their specialisms, including sociology.

Lesbian scholars have been strongly influenced by feminism, which has enabled the development of a more rigorous and sophisticated critique than that developed by gay men (Plummer 1992). The naturalising of gender roles and the relations of power of heteropatriarchal society were first critiqued and deconstructed by feminists (gender being more obviously oppressive to women than to queers), which gave rise to a politicised and sophisticated deconstructionist approach to gendered sexual identities and the sociology of the erotic. A feminist approach, based on a critique of the cultural and social constructions complicit in the subordination of women, is able to support a more rigorous and critical theorising of heterosexual hegemony than the liberal/liberatory approach of traditional gay liberation. In this context it is perhaps unsurprising that it is a woman, Eve Kosofsky Sedgwick, who has developed the most far-reaching and influential reading of the nature and function of the homo/hetero (sexual) binary in modern Western culture (Sedgwick 1985, 1991), a reading described by Plummer as 'feminist gay male theory' (Plummer 1992: 9), and another woman, Judith Butler, who is currently at the forefront of theorising the links between gender and sexuality.

THE PROBLEM OF HOMOSEXUALITY OR THE PROBLEM OF HETEROSEXISM?

This new concern with refocusing the debate away from the assumedly problematic 'homosexuality' and on to the wider area of sexual identity and the place of the erotic in society, represented the beginnings of a significant paradigm shift within sociology. Ken Plummer describes this shift as starting with a 'turning away from a focus on the phenomenon of homosexuality to the mechanics of role constitution and its effect on individuals' and called for an 'ethnography of societal reactions to same-sex experiences' (Plummer 1981a). In other words, the shift in focus begins with a new interest, not in homosexuality itself but rather in how society at large constructs homosexuality, how the label is deployed, and the impact of this on homosexuals and heterosexuals and on homosexuality as a category.

Further impetus was given by social historians such as Jeffrey Weeks, John d'Emilio and Jonathan Katz, whose work involved the study of lesbian and gay people, communities and circumstances in the recent or more distant historical past. Such an enterprise inevitably requires that the categories 'lesbian' and 'gay' themselves be recognised as problematic, as fluid and contingent rather than as describing fixed types of people to be found at all times and in all places. From such work developed an entirely new set of questions about the social factors which make it possible and/or necessary to categorise people according to their sexual preference: 'What made it possible for eroticism to become the basis for an identity that some people took on?' (d'Emilio 1983). Clearly, once this stage has been reached, then it is sexual identity *per se*, and the political and social significance attached to it, which is the focus of inquiry. This means that heterosexuality and the institutions which support it (such as marriage, different kinship and family arrangements, religious beliefs) are dethroned from their invisible and unquestioned position as hegemonic norm and themselves become problematic: the paradigmatic shift is in place.

It must not be imagined that this shift has rocked the foundations of mainstream sociology. Sexuality is still a marginal and stigmatised area of research, and no doubt there are as many heterosexist and homophobic individuals within sociology as in any other field. Sociology, moreover, is still negotiating its status as a 'real' science (Giddens 1989), and is leery, therefore, of being seen to encourage work which might be seen as political or 'unscientific'. However, the deconstruction of both gender and sexuality have been influential within sociology to an extent not echoed in, for example, psychology (Kitzinger 1990, 1991), and this offers some optimism that a lesbian-positive sociology may be a realistic option.

The nature of feminism as an ethical (as well as a political) set of debates has also been influential in the development of a characteristically lesbian-feminist position, and this has informed lesbian research and writing in the social sciences.

LESBIAN SOCIOLOGY, FEMINISM AND WOMEN'S STUDIES

As Plummer (1992) points out, until the advent of HIV/AIDS, there was no natural 'home' for gay men's studies. The availability of relatively generous funding for HIV/AIDS-related research has resulted in an expansion of sociological investigation into the lives of gay men, something not shared by lesbians (as the group least at risk from the sexual transmission of HIV infection in these early days of the epidemic in the developed world). The implications of funding for research being linked to an association of male homosexuality with disease, and to a focus on gay men specifically as a *sexual* minority, are many and complex and deserve urgent study. It is probably not too far fetched to suggest that differences between lesbians and gay men are likely to be exacerbated by the positioning of lesbians alongside feminism and women's studies and the positioning of gay men alongside studies in epidemiology, sexual behaviour, sexual risk and the generally vicious social opprobrium attendant on the epidemic.[3]

Lesbian sociology has shifted focus from a desire on the part of heterosexuals to understand lesbianism as pathology or alien lifestyle, through a changed desire on the part of heterosexuals to understand lesbians as an oppressed minority, to a desire on the part of lesbians themselves to develop and disseminate accounts of lesbianism to further the social, political and psychological needs of a lesbian community. Within the academy, its intellectual debt to feminism means that its natural 'home' is within women's studies. But what is it? Can there be a specifically lesbian praxis within sociology, or must lesbianism be understood merely as as object of sociological enquiry?

TOWARDS A LESBIAN SOCIOLOGICAL PRAXIS

Part of the core problem for lesbian studies, as for women's studies, is the intransigent object-status of lesbian (*qua* sexual deviant and qua woman) within social science discourse. A foregrounding of lesbian scholarship rather than of lesbian-ness as object of enquiry requires that we consider not only how lesbian-ness and lesbian issues may be investigated and presented from a lesbian perspective but also how an identified and avowedly lesbian perspective may be properly and productively focused on *all* topics. What might constitute a lesbian sociological perspective or a set of lesbian research and writing practices? How may/should non-lesbian researchers adapt their research methods? What makes a lesbian sociologist different from other sociologists and is a lesbian praxis possible?

There are two important strands in the development of a lesbian sociology. The first is closely related to the on-going debates concerning the characteristics of a feminist epistemology/methodology and, as such, is probably familiar in outline if not in detail. The second concerns the disputed (and hence disruptive) status of lesbian-ness itself and the implications of that status for the practice of sociology generally.

Feminist praxis (and this is a debate which has been sited almost exclusively within the social sciences, specifically sociology and social policy) has been characterised by Liz Stanley as reflexive, democratic and concerned with the (gendered and inequitable) relations of production in the 'academic mode of production' (Stanley 1990). Feminist researchers are likely to favour qualitative over quantitative methodology, though there is a clear political imperative to make use of whatever methods and techniques are appropriate to investigate, theorise and (by implication) improve the social position of women (Stanley and Wise 1979, Stanley 1990). There is general agreement among feminist sociologists that the researcher has a responsibility to 'account for the conditions of . . . production' of the research, to relate epistemology to 'feminist ontology' and, reflexively, to pay attention to the interactionist process of the research itself. In other words, a feminist research praxis should avoid replicating the hierarchical relations of power which feminism has criticised and should at least be consonant with (if not actively furthering of) the political goals of feminism.

Clearly not all lesbians are feminist, and it would be wrong to assume that feminist epistemological/methodological strategies are necessarily appropriate for a lesbian sociology. What feminist social science has developed, however, is an epistemology disobedient to the power relations inherent in what Patricia Hill Collins calls 'the Eurocentric, masculinist knowledge validation process' (Collins 1990: 203). It is a praxis which foregrounds issues of power and privilege, mandates reflexivity on the part of the researcher, and accepts the contingent and political nature of 'truth'. As such, it has much to offer as an epistemology of resistance and has been adopted and customised in the production of Black sociology (Collins 1990) and lesbian and gay sociology (Faraday 1981) among others. In addition, it incorporates a sensitivity to gender dynamics which is clearly useful to lesbian research although, in common with other feminist scholarship, feminist sociology too often fails to interrogate related issues of sexuality and the erotic. I suggest that feminism has done the epistemological groundwork on which a more finely-tuned lesbian sociology would do well to build, whether or not it subscribes to a feminist ontology.

It is essential, too, that a lesbian sociology refuses to fall into the trap of becoming as white and Eurocentric as the malestream praxis it is attempting to displace. Lesbians of colour are a particularly vulnerable group, subject to race, class and gender oppression as well as homophobia. Homophobia is particularly damaging when it originates within the very communities in which Black lesbians seek collective support against racism, as Barbara Smith points out:

The oppression that affects Black gay people, female and male, is pervasive, constant and not abstract. Some of us die from it. . . . What I think many heterosexual Black people don't know, and don't want to know, is the toll homophobia takes on a daily basis. Too many pretend that lesbian and gay oppression is an inconsequential matter, not a real oppression.

(Collins 1990: 192–3)

Being white in the West is as much an unexamined norm as being heterosexual, while racism intersects powerfully with heterosexism (and with class) in ways which impact on white lesbians as much as on lesbians of colour. If white privilege and 'whiteness' remain unproblematic within lesbian sociology it will remain as limited and, ultimately, anachronistic (and racist) as heterosexist sociology.

LESBIAN SOCIOLOGY FOR NON-LESBIAN SOCIOLOGISTS

Just as not all lesbians are feminist, not all feminist researchers are lesbian and not all politically aware and anti-oppressive researchers are feminist: indeed, many are men and hence debarred (*pace*, Queer Nation!) from becoming lesbian at all. How should a lesbian sociological praxis influence non-lesbian research? My answer is that this probably parallels the (as yet incomplete) paradigmatic shift consequent on 'writing women in' (Pascal 1986). By 'writing lesbians in' to sociology the operations of the heterosexual imperative become apparent. By refusing to assume heterosexuality (especially in women, whose identity within social scientific discourse continues to be constituted in relation to men) and by recognising the existence of a lesbian alternative *in all social contexts*, sociologists may develop a praxis which is more entire, more finely tuned and more alert to the specifics of power. On the other hand, to continue to ignore lesbian possibility results not only in an untruthful, unrepresentative sociology but also in a much diminished, naive, partial and often entirely inappropriate intellectual grasp of social life. The much vaunted sociological imagination is profoundly restricted by unexamined heterosexism/homophobia, as it still is, of course, by unexamined sexism/misogyny (Abbott and Wallace 1990) and racism. Opening up sociology to lesbian possibility promises to enrich and enlighten the discipline immeasurably.

Lesbian sociology offers in its turn crucially important insights for feminism. A good example of this is Gill Dunne's research into 'non-heterosexual' women's perceptions of work (Dunne 1992). Liberal and socialist feminism both have critiques of women's unequal position in the labour market (see Charles and other writers in Feminist Review Collective 1986) and both make links between the domestic division of labour and women's restricted access to paid labour. Yet both have stopped short of an analysis which identifies heterosexuality as a significant factor in the equation. Anti-discrimination and equal pay legislation have not made many inroads into the structural subordination of women in the labour market, and research such as Dunne's, which seems to show quite clearly that rejecting heterosexuality leads to a greatly improved career picture for women (Dunne 1992), offers an important new approach to a problem which is clearly not going to be solved by legislation alone. If heterosexual women's orientation towards marriage is one factor inhibiting equal access to the labour market (as Dunne's research suggests), then political strategies which aim to emancipate women as a class need to incorporate this understanding if they are to succeed. This is only one example of the potential benefits of a lesbian sociology for non-lesbians.

Oppression is not the sole defining characteristic of lesbians. Rather, membership of an oppressed minority is the *modern paradigm* for lesbian existence, the definitional imperative of identity. Lesbian identity must be understood as specifically modern, rather than as something always and already existing outwith the realm of the textual and the discursive. The implications of this for lesbian sociology are both powerful and potentially paralysing. Recognition of the contingent and constructed nature of lesbian identity exposes the equally contingent and constructed nature of heterosexuality, the social (rather than biological or psychological) nature of sexual desire and practice and (by implication) the contingent, constructed and inherently political nature of other modern organisational categories such as blackness, whiteness, youth, etc. (see [charles] 1992, Rutherford 1990, Ware 1992). The potential for paralysis lies in the self-deconstructive paradox of lesbian studies – or of any set of activities predicated upon the presumed ontological stability of a taxonomic category which is, in fact, contingent and permeable. It is only by the now familiar device of naming 'lesbian' as strategic rather than ontological that we may validate the coherence of a lesbian sociology.

A lesbian sociology is one among many interventions within the academic sphere which enable a radical revisioning of the social – a paradigmatic shift curiously akin to the new physics of chaos and string theory. Identifying 'lesbian' as discursively produced also exposes the partial, constitutive (rather than descriptive, explorative) and political nature of academic discourse (Plummer 1992). Sociology itself, as a paradigm, is up for grabs within this set of 'postmodern queeries'. Problematising sexual identity and gender may be seen as among the first practices which lead to the rejection of the metanarrative characteristic of post modernity,[4] and sociology is just such a one.

A lesbian sociology may perhaps be characterised by a willingness to engage with the small scale, the temporary, the fragmentary; to work with the understanding that an attempt to construct any kind of unifying grand design out of the multiple and contradictory social moments which are lesbian and gay lives and groupings (which are, indeed, the seemingly monolithic homophobias and heterosexisms of different hegemonic social and cultural groupings) is not so much doomed to failure as intrinsically flawed and misconceived. Such insights first developed within cultural studies but are rapidly making inroads into the social sciences (see, for example, Game 1991) and have already made their lively and disobedient presence felt in the lesbian and gay social sciences. It is no accident that British sociologist Ken Plummer has titled his recent edited collection *Modern Homosexualities: Fragments of Lesbian and Gay Experience* (1992), a telling departure from his earlier collection, *The Making of the Modern Homosexual* (1981b).

LESBIAN SOCIETY

In conclusion I would like to set a tentative agenda for lesbian sociological research. The social life of lesbians has been largely ignored in mainstream sociology. There are also interesting questions concerning the impact of wider social and demographic change on lesbians and lesbian groups. For example, most commentators agree that a specific combination of economic and demographic circumstances consequent on the Industrial Revolution made it possible for women to *be* what we now think of as 'lesbian' (d'Emilio and Freedman 1988, Faderman 1981, 1991). The taxonomic activity identified by Foucault as catalysing the birth of the homosexual 'species' was not in itself sufficient to enable women to become part of that species, material change was also necessary.

The break up of tightly knit agrarian communities and the mass urban migration which marked the historical beginnings of industrial capitalism influenced the development of lesbian identity in specific ways. Waged labour enabled women to work outside the domestic sphere, giving them an emotional and economic independence inconceivable in earlier times. The consequent shift in gender relations and the spreading secularisation of society loosened the moral and economic bonds which had so ruthlessly limited women's options. As households shrank from the large extended family of the agrarian economy to the modern 'nuclear' model, streamlined in order to reproduce the labour force and to provide a ready market for consumer goods, it became viable for two women to set up and run a household together. More recent changes – liberalisation of the divorce laws, an increase in women's earning power, the growth of the Welfare State and the commodification of goods and services – have meant that, probably for the first time in history, marriage is an *option* rather than a necessity for the majority of women in the industrial nations (though it is important to recognise that this is far from so for women in much of the developing world). If your children go to school from the age of four, if you can purchase food rather than having to grow it, if there are minimal state benefits to support you before your children reach school age, then your survival no longer depends on marriage. The implications for lesbians, and indeed for theories of sexual identity, are profound. For if heterosexual marriage has become a choice so, too, has lesbian-ness.

Social history and demography are not, of course, the only areas of interest to lesbian sociology. Research into key sociological issues – questions of stigma, of deviance, of labelling, of discrimination and of sub-cultural formation – have all tended in the past to ignore lesbians. Yet the experience of lesbians is an important source of information in all these areas. There are, additionally, things which sociology has to offer which are of importance to lesbians. An investigation into the differences between rural and urban lesbians is long overdue. Most lesbian sub-cultural activity is assumed to be urban in nature and to revolve around clubs and pubs, telephone helplines and discos. This assumption motivates a queer migration to major cities in the West, a migration which in itself gives rise to many potential problems. Yet there *are* rural lesbian communities (see, for example, Stokes 1985), although published information about them is sparse. Comparative research into urban and rural lesbian communities is, in fact, essential if we are to develop a sophisticated model of sexual identity, to broaden our meanings of 'lesbian' beyond the stereotype of the urban bar scene so familiar from lesbian novels, or to establish effective and appropriate support for young and 'new' lesbians. That so many inexperienced and vulnerable lesbians are drawn to strange cities in the search for their peers should be of concern to the community as a whole.

The invisibility of rural lesbians is but one consequence of the erasure of lesbian existence from the social world more generally. Lesbian sociology has a major part to play in filling in the gaps in our social knowledge and, in so doing, will enrich not only the practice of sociology but also the lives of lesbians and of lesbian communities. Wherever you look, mainstream sociology is weakened by its failure to recognise lesbian possibility, and lesbians are weakened by being denied information about who we are and the different solutions we have devised to the problem of living on what I have elsewhere called 'Planet Hetero' (Wilton 1993b: 275). Research into changing forms of lesbian family and household, into the social position of lesbians and lesbian households within different ethnic communities and different socio-economic milieu, into the social construction of gender within lesbian and gay communities as compared to the heterosexual mainstream, these are but a few of the neglected and exciting areas where lesbian sociology could have much to offer both sociology and lesbians.

NOTES

1 Of course, male homosexual activity *was* criminal at this time in Britain and the United States, which may partly explain the concern with male as opposed to female homosexuality, since homosexuals were part of the criminal underclass which so intrigued early sociologists.

2 Of course, using autobiographical accounts does not of itself imply equality between researcher and researched (see discussions in Stanley 1990). However, when such equity is among the aims of the research, autobiography is a particularly apposite method.

3 That these differences are already the source of painful conflict between lesbians and some gay men is clear from the heated debate sparked by the remarks of gay British AIDS commentator Simon Watney on Channel 4's lesbian and gay magazine programme 'Out'. Watney said that he found the demands of lesbians for information and support around HIV issues 'insulting to gay men', and the response in the gay press revealed both deep-seated antagonisms between lesbians and gay men and a widespread failure of the 'lesbian-and-gay community' to take women's issues on board (see, for example, Collis 1992, Ross 1992, Watney 1992).

4 Of course, this type of deconstruction work has its roots in feminist writing of an extraordinarily early time. From Mary Wollstonecraft through Simone de Beauvoir up to contemporary writers such as Judith Butler, gender has been problematised and recognised as constructed by social factors in the interests of the ruling class of men. Lesbian and gay theory has thus developed out of a long tradition within feminist theory.

Chapter 9

Subject to control
Lesbians and the state

Citizenship is a problematic and contested concept and it is particularly so for women. For lesbians, whose sexuality is publicly anathematised and whose incorporation in the group 'women' is for various reasons far from straightforward, citizenship bears little relation to that taken for granted by most people in contemporary liberal democracies.

The notion of citizenship includes obligations and benefits. Unsurprisingly, it assumes that the citizen is male. The paradigmatic citizen is the soldier, whose duty is to die for his nation when necessary. During the struggle for women's suffrage in Britain the chief argument against allowing women the vote was that, since they could not fight in war, according them citizenship would place the state in jeopardy (Pateman 1992). In Britain, where the symbolic residue of monarchy holds sway and where there is no written constitution to guarantee individual rights, the question is further muddied by the fact that the political status of the people is that of 'subject' rather than 'citizen'. This does not alter the key fact that women are excluded from the classic concept of citizenship:

> [C]itizenship has been constructed in the male image. Women, our bodies and distinctive capacities, represented all that citizenship and equality are not. 'Citizenship' has gained its meaning through the exclusion of women, that is to say (sexual) difference.
>
> (Pateman 1992: 19)

Pateman goes on to explain that there is one way for women to attain a limited kind of citizenship. For women the ultimate duty lies in motherhood, in *reproducing* the state. And it is here, clearly, that one central problem for lesbians is located. Lesbians share to a certain extent the position of all women in relation to the state. On the other hand, such benefits as do accrue to women through citizenship and especially through membership of a Welfare State, depend by and large on a woman's 'proper' relationship with *a man*. It is as mothers *within a heterosexual family unit* that women are allowed full state benefits (including widow's pension, for example) and a recognised, albeit limited, citizenship. Adult lesbians, as women existing on the outside of male-headed domesticity, and in particular as women who render problematic the relationship between femaleness and maternity (either by not mothering, or by mothering outside a heterosexual dyad), simply do not fit into any social policy slot.

GENDER, MOTHERING AND THE STATE

The complex relationship between women, mothering and the state tends to render meaningless common-sense assumptions about the division between the public and the private spheres. On the one hand, it is by becoming a mother that a woman achieves a place in the socio-political order. 'Motherhood as a political status, as a major vehicle of women's incorporation into the political order, has shaped women's duty to the state and women's citizenship' (Pateman 1992: 22). On the other hand, it is precisely *because* of their ability to mother that women's bodies (and their political and social selves) have been so rigidly controlled within all patriarchal political systems.

Recent attempts by the British Government to restrict unmarried women's access to donated sperm enforce heterosexual compliance as the price of motherhood. This is not new; the male state has long attempted to control women's reproductivity (Corea 1985). And, just as the men expended in the nation-state's warmaking are ranked by colour and class, so too are the women who reproduce the state. Whilst white middle-class women have been urged to do their reproductive duty, minority ethnic women, working-class, Jewish, disabled or intellectually impaired women have all been variously prevented from conceiving or bearing children.

Thus, in the early twentieth century in Australia, childless (white) women were castigated as 'a menace to social purity and national stability', while in the USA President Roosevelt declared them to be contemptible cowards, comparing them to a man who 'fears to do his duty in battle when the country calls him' (Pateman 1992). The other side of this eugenicist coin is the enforced sterilisation/abortion of women deemed inferior. The familiar 'racial hygiene' practices of the German Third Reich were but the most blatant example of widespread, state-enforced atrocities designed to maintain racial purity. When the Nazis sterilised and aborted millions of women – Jews, Romanies,

Slavs, the disabled and intellectually impaired – this was war crime, but in the United States the officially sanctioned, compulsory sterilisation of Black, Native American and Latina women went on well into the second half of the twentieth century. The racist abuse of sterilisation or long-term contraceptive techniques is still taking place in the industrialised West and the Third World (Berer 1984, Davis 1982). In former Yugoslavia as I write, Serbian 'ethnic cleansing' strategies include the forcible impregnation of Bosnian Moslem women by Serb soldiers (Pitter and Stiglmayer 1993), while the genocidal policies of China in Tibet include preventing Tibetan women having children.

Wherever a nation-state or a dominant 'race' feels itself under threat, it intervenes in the child-bearing of women. What we may naïvely believe to be a private and profoundly personal decision, whether or not to conceive and bear a child, is in fact utterly and blatantly at the whim of governments, whether democratic or despotic:

> [T]he Ceausescu regime in Romania enforced women's duty in the harshest fashion to try to attain a population of 30 million at the end of the twentieth century, banning contraception and abortion and policing women workers to ensure that all pregnancies were detected and brought to term.
>
> (Pateman 1992: 25).

Women achieve citizenship – and sometimes it is thrust upon them – through their reproductive allegiance to the state. At the same time, their reproductivity is closely controlled by the state (and of course by many patriarchal religions, especially when these are religions of the state such as in Catholic Ireland or Muslim Pakistan). Giving birth is more an obligation than a right of the female citizen and, as such, is inextricably linked to the socio-political status of the woman concerned. In the West, reproduction is most certainly the obligation (and hence the right) of white, middle-class, able-bodied women. The 'right' to conceive and give birth is often denied to disabled, working class or minority women in the interests of eugenicist ideologies implicit in the very idea of the nation state. Through childbirth, then, women are subject to very direct state control.

Where does this leave lesbians? Along with gypsies and prostitutes, lesbians were exterminated as social undesirables in Hitler's death camps (Haeberle 1989). Most groups consigned to the Final Solution are still oppressed in the West today and lesbians are no exception. The contemporary nation-state, organised as it is around a gendered division of power and labour (and dependent upon that division) is by definition an oppressor of women. For women who are lesbians, and who therefore transgress (if not actually transcend) that division, it has no place. In some ways, being outcast from the body politic is a liberating position, in many more ways it is a uniquely dangerous place to be. This chapter attempts to outline the peculiarities which comprise lesbian citizenship and the effect of social policy upon lesbians. It includes discussion of a broad range of social policy issues including income support, welfare, education, healthcare, housing, parenting, policing and youth and community work. Again, this really requires an entire book, and all that is possible here is a superficial skim over the surface.

WELFARE, FAMILIES AND THE INVISIBLE DYKE

Social policy, by definition, directly affects everyone living under any kind of formal political structure. Its impact on individuals varies according to their social status, their material circumstances, their access to resources and the degree of control they have over their lives. To a large extent, lesbians share the social and material status of all women, but with significant and usually unrecognised differences.

The social status of women globally, although culturally and geographically contingent, is inferior to that of men (Morgan 1984, New Internationalist 1985, Seager and Olson 1986). There are important local differences in the symbolic, material, organisational and political structures of patriarchal power, but such structures weigh on women around the planet. Relative to men, women are kept poor, unhealthy, uneducated and powerless, and lesbians share in that general disadvantage.

Although sexuality and sexual identity are differently shaped and differently experienced within disparate (and sometimes incomparable) cultural, social and geographic locations, homosexuality exists world-wide and is subject to a variety of social, legal and physical restraints and punishments (The Pink Book Editing Team 1988, Weinrich and Williams 1991). Lesbians share in some sense the social position 'homosexual' with gay men, though this positioning is modulated by the interventions of gender and, in particular, of male power and male economic advantage. It is impossible in this short space to present a global analysis. What follows is an assessment of the position of lesbians within the British Welfare State, though much of what I say will be recognised in the context of most so-called First World countries, all of which have some variety of welfare provision, and has relevance to much of what goes on in the countries of the former Soviet Union.

WOMEN AND CHILDREN FIRST – WELFARE FOR THE SONS OF EMPIRE

The origins of the British Welfare State are rooted in the militaristic, expansionist foreign policy of colonialism. Many significant welfare initiatives followed on the heels of war. The chronic poor health of recruits for the Boer War lead to the focus on maternal and child health which so dominated early welfare provision, and the propaganda needs consequent on the Second World War (the notion that a 'land fit for heroes' must be offered as sufficient justification for a war increasingly questioned by pacifists and involving civilians on a scale previously unknown) hastened the setting up of a National Health Service and comprehensive benefit system (Ham 1992). Also influential was the historical involvement of charitable and philanthropic interests motivated by moral and religious doctrine. This strand resulted in the distinction between the 'deserving' and the 'undeserving' poor and in the imposition of middle-class ideas and standards of behaviour on the working class. It also resulted in the policing of sexual behaviour, specifically women's sexual behaviour. Much early protective legislation concerning the working conditions of women and children, as well as such measures as the infamous Contagious Diseases Act of 1864, were motivated by a desire to restrain working-class (hetero)sexual activity (Wells 1982). Ironically, much early feminist work took much the same line: the nineteenth-century women's movement in both the UK and the USA (Ehrenreich and English 1973, d'Emilio and Freedman 1988, Hobson 1987) was allied to temperance and 'social purity', which was largely a euphemism for sexual restraint.

The end result of this historical process was a Welfare State organised around the idea of women's dependency (Pascal 1986) and services which both assumed and maintained the centrality of motherhood in women's lives and identities (and, hence, the secondary status of women's own needs). Women are primarily defined within social policy discourse by their role as carers, a role seen as economically non-productive, despite the dependence of the capitalist state on this body of unpaid labour. The extent to which the Welfare State depends on women's unpaid caring work (of young children, male partners and elderly dependent relatives) has been revealed in recent years (Equal Opportunities Commission 1982a, 1982b, 1984), and socialist feminists have argued for recognition of the material contribution to capitalist production of women's unwaged labour in reproducing and maintaining the labour force (Beechey 1978, Pascal 1986).

WAGED LABOUR

Women find themselves in a vicious circle. Because of their domestic and caring responsibilities they have a discontinuous relationship to the labour market, usually returning to work on a lower-paid, lower-status and often part-time basis after raising children and often having to leave paid work at an early age to care for elderly relatives. Women whose lives are not organised around heterosexual family life – including many lesbians – are affected by the structural inequalities which have developed around the assumption that domestic work is women's primary role. Among these structural inequalities are the notion of the male 'family wage' as against women's 'pin money' and the belief that a man makes a better employee than a woman since he will not take time off work to give birth or care for sick children. Thus, the assumption that a woman's place is in the (heterosexual) home results in women experiencing poor working conditions, lower pay and discrimination outside the home. This, in turn, helps to ensure that their paid work is seen as of secondary importance in the heterosexual family and justifies them being lumbered with an unequal share of domestic labour within the home . . . which makes it impossible for them to join the labour market on equal terms, and so the cycle continues.

Some writers have seen it as an aspect of lesbian oppression that lesbians have much less choice than heterosexual women about whether or not they participate in waged labour:

> Lesbians must work. Put most simply, few lesbians will ever have, however briefly, the economic support of another person . . . lesbians are dependent on themselves for subsistence. Thus, a significant portion of the time and energies of most lesbians is devoted to working.
>
> (Schneider 1984: 211)

On the other hand, there are undoubted *some* economic advantages for women in rejecting heterosexuality: the interrupted career pattern caused by having and caring for children obviously penalises women, and the assumption that entry to the labour market is a temporary measure pending marriage deprives women of a realistic assessment of their career options and abilities (Dunne 1992). Yet these advantages are apparent rather than real for most lesbians. First, there are many 'invisible' economic benefits to heterosexual marriage which are not available to lesbians. State and company pension schemes do not apply to same-sex couples, something which is starting to concern unions. NALGO (the National Association of Local Government Officers), for example, published a statement from the lesbian and gay lobbying group Stonewall to the effect that, 'same-sex couples in public sector super-annuation schemes are subsidising married members, since they pay the same contributions but get worse benefits' (Moriarty 1993). Second, while Dunne's research shows that a non-heterosexual orientation to the labour market is advantageous for women it does not obviate the effects of gender. Lesbians may not escape from the pre-existing inequalities of the labour market. Women earn less than men and have a much narrower range of work options open to them, and although lesbians may or may not earn on average more than heterosexual women (and the research has not yet been done which would enable us to say whether they do or not), they still earn less than men.

In addition, the supposed advantage of non-heterosexuality presumes that non-heterosexual is synonymous with 'non-mother'. Many lesbians have children, and the children of a lesbian need just as much care and hence represent just as much of a disadvantage in the labour market as the children of a non-lesbian. Yet again, although many lesbians have been lesbian since adolescence, many others have not. It is very common for lesbians to have spent many years in heterosexual relationships before becoming lesbian, and for these women we may not assume a 'non-heterosexual' orientation to the labour market at that crucial early point in their working lives.

For gay men, whose *masculinity* gives them an advantage in the labour market to start with, their *sexuality* may bring both advantage and disadvantage. Although they are less likely than heterosexual men to have economic responsibility for children, there is no employment protection for lesbians and gay men and they risk job loss if their sexual identity becomes known at their place of work. Although, for a minority of lesbians, their *sexuality* may go some way towards offsetting the disadvantage of their gender, for most this is probably not significant relative to the profound disadvantage women suffer in the labour market *as* women, and the lack of job security they experience as lesbians is an added disadvantage. To be queer and female is, in economic terms, little different from being straight and female, but the social implications are significant. Given the desperate need for solidarity and for community when faced with the daily humiliations and dangers of living in a hostile culture, the unquestioned male dominance of the gay sub-culture is a very real problem for many lesbians.

WELFARE AND THE LESBIAN CITIZEN

Benefit entitlement, pension rights, housing policy and education all assume (and act to ensure) women's dependency on men and the primacy of their role as mothers (Pascal 1986). The assumption that women's welfare matters primarily insofar as it affects their ability to mother the nation's children runs explicitly through Beveridge's plans for social security. Writing in 1942 the report which was to lay the foundations for the Welfare State, Beveridge was in no doubt of what the purpose of women was:

> In the next thirty years housewives as mothers have vital work to do in ensuring the adequate continuance of the British race and of British ideals in the world.
>
> (Beveridge 1942: 53)

The position of women within the discourse of early welfarism is clear, and current practices have not deviated from this ideology. Women within marriage (or cohabiting with a male partner) are not perceived by the state as individuals, as the DHSS regulations for supplementary benefit make clear: 'A husband and wife who live in the same household form a single assessment unit. Only the husband can normally receive benefit (DHSS 1982: 29).

The Welfare State depends upon women's unpaid domestic labour, so it is in the interests of the state that gender roles be unquestioned. It is therefore a feature of the social construction of gender relations of dependency that they have been profoundly naturalised. The supposed 'laws' of nature and the traditional doctrine of the Christian church[1] have been deployed in support of what is in fact a socio-political system. Thus Patrick Jenkin, when he was Secretary of State for Social Services, claimed: 'If the good Lord had intended us all having equal rights to go out to work and to behave equally, you know he really wouldn't have created man and woman' (Coote and Campbell 1987: 87).[2] The naturalness of the domestic division of labour has implications for the forcefulness and effectiveness of gender socialisation. Thus, men may be dependent on their earning ability (in particular their ability to support a family in traditional, manly style) and on their status as skilled workers for their self-esteem *as men* (Cockburn 1983/1991). This in itself is deeply interwoven with the tradition of the family wage which has so dominated industrial relations and trade-union struggle in post-industrial British history (Charles 1986), and means that the British labour movement fought long and hard to obstruct women's entry to the labour market (Boston 1980, Cockburn 1987). In the USA, too, unions and management have traditionally been suspicious and obstructive of women's equal participation in waged labour (Ruskin and Padavic 1988).

A social policy structure founded upon and intended to support a traditional heterosexual division of labour penalises women who are unattached to men and/or who are not mothers. Women's access or lack of access to a male wage determines their access to housing, their standard of living, their relative wealth or poverty, and the degree of control they can exercise over their lives (Pascal 1986). Lacking access to a male wage and with no recognised place in the structures of social security, lesbians are vulnerable to poverty and to homelessness. Research is needed to find out how these factors impact on the lives of lesbians and what policy changes are needed to protect the rights of lesbian citizens. Social policy research seldom recognises that lesbians exist, or confines comment to a single sentence concerning their absence from collected data (for example, Cook and Watt 1993, Graham 1993).

Lesbians with children are dealt with as single parents by the establishment. There is no legal recognition of lesbian partnerships, and few local authorities choose to recognise same-sex couples for tenancy or other purposes. If women have children there is a statutory responsibility on local government to house them, though studies have shown that unmarried mothers (a category which, by default, includes lesbian mothers) are discriminated against in local authority housing practice, often being allocated hard-to-let units, compounding the problems of this especially vulnerable group. There is no understanding (even among gay activist groups) of the implications of such policies for lesbian mothers.

If women with children but without men fare badly, women with neither have little or no claim on welfare services and are pretty much left to fend for themselves. Since many benefits are contributions linked, and since women's earning power is so much less than men's, the safety net of pensions and benefits spectacularly fails never-married women. No research has been carried out, but it is probable that very many elderly lesbians, unable to claim widow's pensions or to benefit from the other financial entitlements which marriage brings, are living in poverty. Again, research singularly fails to recognise their existence – older lesbians are largely absent from mainstream literature (for example, Webb 1993).

LESBIAN WORK – LESBIAN LIVES

Lesbians are subject to double jeopardy under such a frankly discriminatory system. They share with non-lesbian women the problematic relationship to the labour market which has grown out of assumptions about women's domestic role. The end result is a chronic lack of educational and training opportunities, a lower average wage than men, poorer working conditions, an increased likelihood of ending up in part-time, low-status and insecure work, confinement to sterotypically 'feminine' sectors of the labour market and restricted promotion prospects. In addition, lesbian partnerships are seldom recognised by housing authorities or private landlords and never in pensions or insurance rights. A lesbian council tenant whose partner dies may not be entitled automatically to continue the tenancy and lesbians are unlikely to be allocated public housing, other than hard-to-let, and increasingly rare, single-person accommodation. Lesbian couples may find it difficult to get mortgages,[3] impossible to obtain privately rented property, and may find themselves unlikely to be accepted by hard-pressed housing associations. Pensions will reflect the lower earning power a lesbian has as a woman and will not benefit life partners. Lesbians suffer all the consequences of deviating from the familial norm around which social policy has been devised.

LESBIAN MOTHERING

Despite a recent liberalisation of official attitudes to lesbian mothers, they still face the continual threat of losing their children (Allen and Harne 1988, Alpert 1988, Crane 1982, Rights of Women Lesbian Custody Group 1986) and discrimination in housing, healthcare and maternity services, their children's schooling and access to family benefits. There is little recognition of the existence of lesbian mothers in either the heterosexual or the lesbian and gay community, and such mothers may be even more isolated than their heterosexual counterparts. It is significant, for example, that the report of a London conference held in October 1988 by CHAR (the Housing Campaign for Single People) on housing for lesbians and gay men, while discussing lesbians and gays with disabilities, leaving psychiatric instititions, having HIV or leaving care, has no mention of lesbian mothers. Lesbians, too, are more likely than heterosexual women to be estranged from their families of origin (CHAR 1988, London Strategic Policy Unit 1985), and so are likely to lack extended family support during pregnancy and with the care of babies and young children.

The New Right, especially in the UK and the USA, has made political capital out of perceived threats to the family and has constructed and manipulated links between homosexuality, left-wing extremism and godlessness in order to embody and demonise this threat and to mobilise support against it. For a politic which attempts to structure the social arena around an idea of the nation as family, the idea of the homosexual as enemy within – the embodied challenge to the naturalness of familial ideology – is a necessary fiction (Shepherd 1989). If homosexuals did not exist it would have been necessary for the New Right to invent us. And invent us they have done, cleverly cobbling together a veritable Frankenstein's monster, howling in the outermost darkness around the embattled hearth of the Happy Heterosexual Family.

In order to maintain the fiction of the heterosexual family as a place of safety and sanctuary, the myth of the homosexual child molester is deployed. Although (or perhaps even because) it is, overwhelmingly, *heterosexual* men who rape, beat and abuse women and children, and although such abuse largely happens within the 'safety' of the nuclear family (Hague and Malos 1993), it is *homosexuality* which is characterised as dangerous to children (Herek 1991). In the United States, where anti-gay activist Anita Bryant's campaign organisation *Save Our Children* has done much to whip up public hysteria about the supposed risk to children posed by homosexual adults, a series of recent legislative moves at state and federal level attempted to prohibit various kinds of contact between lesbians and gays and children – including fostering, adoption and even teaching (see Herek 1991). In Britain, the apotheosis of the demonising of homosexuality came with the passing of Section 28 of the 1988 Local Government Act, and it struck specifically at the lesbian or gay family.

SECTION 28 – PRETEND FAMILIES

The history of events which led up to the eventual passing of Section 28 is one of steadily increasing disempowerment of local authorities in England and Wales by the Thatcher administration. As the Thatcher government imposed its monetarist policies with a single-mindedness never before witnessed in democratic government, a degree of opposition came through Labour-controlled local authorities, especially in the London boroughs and the Greater London Council (GLC). It became a priority of central government to weaken the power-base of local government. Additionally, as the ideological starting point of the New Right administration was an anti-collectivist market liberalism, the small but significant advances which a handful of local authorities had made in the area of equal opportunities was political anathema. For both these reasons, local government equal opportunities policies (especially in the powerful and relatively radical GLC) were singled out for attack.

In 1986, the Conservative Earl of Halsbury introduced a Private Member's Bill, 'An Act to restrain local authorities from promoting homosexuality', in the House of Lords. At the time, the Bill was not popular with the government of the time and was dropped in the run up to the general election. The next year, David Wilshire, one of the Conservative members of the committee debating the Local Government Bill, added the now infamous Section 28 (then Clause 26), broadly based on Halsbury's Bill, and it was adopted by the government. The Section states:

(1) A local authority shall not
  (a) intentionally promote homosexuality or publish material with the intention of promoting homosexuality;
  (b) promote the teaching in any maintained school of the acceptability of homosexuality as a pretended family relationship;
(2) Nothing in subsection (1) above shall be taken to prohibit the doing of anything for the purpose of treating or preventing the spread of disease.

Subsection (2) was, of course, added in order to protect those charged with educating people about HIV/AIDS and, as such, reinforces in British law the unhelpful and offensive link between homosexuality and disease. The main text of the Section is interesting for several reasons and powerfully exposes the ideological construction of 'homosexuality' and 'family' in current circulation.

First, there is the overt heterosexualisation of 'the family'. Lesbians and gay men, within the understanding of this law, cannot have family relationships, they may only 'pretend' to do so. While obviously farcical (lesbians and gay men do not materialise like gods and goddesses from Olympus, we have parents, siblings, grandparents, aunts and uncles in abundance), this sentence enraged British gay men and lesbians in particular. The implication that a lesbian mother may only *pretend* to a family relationship with her child exposes with appalling viciousness the extent to which a homophobic administration is able simply to write homosexuals out of the human race. It also exposes the precariousness of the fiction of the sacred bond between mother and child on which much right-wing propaganda rests.

The second important point revealed by the Section is the assumed nature of same-sex desire. You cannot promote something unless it is *learned behaviour*. And, indeed, many of the debates which raged in both Houses during the progress of the Section through Parliament revolved around just this issue, are homosexuals born or made (Colvin and Hawksely 1989)? The assumption that homosexuality is learned behaviour lies behind most anti-gay legislation. It only makes sense to ban lesbians from teaching in schools or from fostering and adopting children if the assumption is that they are out to 'recruit'.

Whatever the long-term political implications of the apparent consensus within the gay community to fight Section 28 on the essentialist ticket, the short-term political costs of the law being passed have hit deep. Despite being so badly drafted that legal experts have dubbed it 'unworkable' (Colvin and Hawksley 1989), its repercussions have been felt widely, mostly throughout the education system and in youth work. The especial vulnerability of young lesbians and gay men mean that it has been extremely harmful.

QUEER YOUTH – LESBIANS AND THE EDUCATION AND YOUTH SERVICES

Growing up gay can be difficult. For young lesbians, having to struggle with sexism as well as heterosexism and homophobia, it is often doubly hard. Neither the lesbian and gay community, largely located in pubs and clubs and as thoroughly male-dominated as the straight world, nor mainstream schools and youth clubs, are safe and supportive places for young lesbians (Harris 1990, Trenchard 1989, Trenchard and Warren 1984). Schoolchildren use sexist and homophobic abuse from a surprisingly early age to police peer behaviour (Mahony 1989), and research done in the United States reveals not only that there is widespread violence against lesbian and gay students in state schools and colleges, but that, 'while evidence shows serious problems for many groups, the most severe hostilities are directed against lesbians and gay men' (Berrill 1990 in Norris 1992). Educational institutions are hostile and dangerous places for young lesbians. For adult lesbians, a career in education or youthwork may be isolating or risky. Because of the widely promulgated myth that lesbians are out to seduce all girl children and young women, being open as a lesbian is simply impossible for most teachers, residential social workers or youth and community workers.

Many lesbian and gay adults have put energy and dedication into setting up support systems for young people. The shameful statistics on attempted suicide among young lesbians and gay men (and some, of course, succeed) shows the urgent need for this kind of work. It is, therefore, in education and in youth and community work that many of the most important initiatives aimed at providing services for lesbians have been situated, and it was at precisely such successful and important work that Section 28 was directed.

Schools are not good places to be female, let alone lesbian. The educational system fails girls in important ways. Their academic ability is consistently underrated and they are directed to employment well below their abilities, the assumption being that employment will be a temporary measure between school and marriage (Griffin 1987, Stanworth 1987). Boys are regarded by teachers as more important and more interesting than girls, the curriculum is geared to boys' interests (Clarricoates 1987, Kessler *et al.* 1987), and both male pupils and male teachers keep female pupils and female teachers in subordination by sexual harassment (Walkerdine 1987). The 'hidden curriculum'[4] of schooling is to maintain the hegemonic division of labour along gender lines. For young gay men the policing of heterosexual masculinity which takes place in schools can be torturous. For young lesbians, treated as second class on the basis of their gender in addition to all the problems associated with their sexuality, the experience can be appalling (Trenchard and Warren 1984). For young lesbians of colour, racism interacts with homophobia and sexism, leading to specific problems.

One spur for Section 28 (following on as it did from an earlier Bill which mentioned schools specifically) was the small but growing body of work being done in a few British schools to meet the needs of lesbian and gay pupils. As long ago as September 1974 the London Gay Teachers' Group (GTG) was formed and in 1986, after a series of battles with (among others), the National Union of Teachers (NUT) and the Inner London Education Authority (ILEA), the first National Conference on lesbian and gay issues in education, jointly organised by GTG and Lesbians in Education, was held. Ironically, it was the ILEA, subsequently to bear the brunt of the Conservative administration's wrath for its equal opportunities work, which in 1974 attracted a lot of publicity for sacking teacher John Warburton for coming out to his pupils in response to questioning. The ILEA chief inspector formally rescinded his dismissal in 1982, explicitly recognising the right of openly gay teachers to teach in ILEA schools. ILEA was also at first openly hostile to the GTG, banning it from meeting on its premises or advertising in its newsletter until 1981 (Gay Teacher's Group 1987). Subsequently, GTG became a valuable resource for lesbian and gay teachers, setting up a helpline, publishing suggested resources for use in classroom discussions of homosexuality and ensuring that the NUT adopted a policy which supported the rights of lesbian and gay teachers.

It is teachers who are themselves lesbian or gay who have taken the initiative not only in setting up support and advocacy systems for their lesbian and gay colleagues, but also in identifying and demanding recognition of the needs of lesbian and gay pupils/students. From heterosexual educationalists there has been little sign of interest or involvement beyond raising a hand to vote for an equal opportunities measure at union conferences. In Britain, there is no equivalent to the Hetrick-Martin Institute for the Protection of Gay and Lesbian Youth and no likelihood of any such support being possible in the forseeable future.

The problems specific to lesbians in schools have, unsurprisingly, been most thoroughly identified and challenged within a lesbian feminist context. Heterosexual feminist research has ignored the specific needs of lesbian teachers and students fairly thoroughly (see, for example Arnot and Weiner 1987, Weiner and Arnot 1987). Within a lesbian feminist paradigm, the experience of heterosexism and sexism which burdens young lesbians is seen as a coherent whole (Jones and Mahony 1989). Within this paradigm, many seemingly disparate problems facing lesbians in schools fall into place as logical outcomes of the patriarchal imperative to retain control of both women and men by stringent policing of gender-appropriate behaviour and to maintain, in particular, the subordination of women. Issues such as the ubiquity of heterosexism within the school regime, the attempt by central government to dictate the content and terms of sex education and HIV/AIDS education, or the impact of Section 28, fall within the remit of feminist theory and political action (see articles by Jackson, Melia, Sanders and Spraggs, and Scott in Jones and Mahony 1989). Outwith a feminist analysis, the traditional sexual-libertarian approach most commonly adopted by gay male political activists is limited to liberal pluralism. Liberalism, while it defends individual freedoms from beaurocratic intervention, is unable to account for the dynamic of gender, or for the interaction between the structural/instititional operation of heterosexism and the psycho-social complexities of homophobia. Some of the pioneering work done by the GLC and ILEA draws its strength and political consistency from its attempts to draw together the threads of sexism and heterosexism.

Further links between other forms of oppression were tentatively made by the Positive Images Group in Harringey between 1986 and 1988. The work of this pioneering group linked racism, heterosexism and sexism, and stressed consultation with local community groups over equal opportunities policies in schools (Cooper 1989). It was in Harringey that the picture book *Jenny Lives with Eric and Martin* was to cause such a furore, when Kenneth Baker (then Secretary of State for Education) announced that as a parent he could not stand by while Harringey allowed the use of such books in schools.

The carefully orchestrated hysteria mounted swiftly, its many idiocies culminating in a press statement from Tottenham Conservative Party condemning Harringey's lesbian and gay unit as 'a greater threat to family life than Adolf Hitler' (Cooper 1987a). The analogy is telling. Not only is there the familiar embodiment of homosexuality as a risk to the family but we are also to understand that our *national* life is in peril. It is only within the context of the nation/family elision that this reference to Hitler may be understood, since of course the policies of the Third Reich were explicitly pro-family and grounded in the idealised, pure, Aryan family.

Education, more openly than any other element of the Welfare State, has a political and ideological function – to produce right-thinking citizens. It is hardly surprising then that not only should the needs of lesbian students and teachers go unrecognised within the education system, but that any attempts to claim equal rights for them should be suppressed with a ruthlessness normally reserved for enemies in wartime. To insist that lesbians have as much right to an education appropriate to their needs and abilities as anyone else is to misunderstand the political nature of the sexual in the contemporary nation state.

YOUTH WORK

Youth and community work is one of the relatively recently professionalised areas within what originated as charitable, philanthropic work done by the middle class for (or to) the disadvantaged. Those who run youth clubs or residential care centres are, increasingly, professionals, with recognised qualifications and membership of professional bodies. The philanthropic origins of youth work are still perceptible in current practice. This can sometimes (though not inevitably) pose severe problems for the services available to young lesbians and gay men, and one dynamic observable in youth work is that between old, established religious values and the newer, professional approach, which stresses equal opportunities and anti-discriminatory practice.

Freer than schools from the stranglehold of central government ideology, youth clubs are often able to do innovative work in 'sensitive' areas such as HIV/AIDS, drugs, racism or sexism, and organisations such as the British Youth Council or Youth Clubs UK have developed a range of excellent materials to support such work. However, sexuality is still an area from which youth workers shy away (Aggleton *et al.* 1990, Davidson 1990), and any discussion of homosexuality is still taboo in most settings involving young people. Section 28 resulted in widespread devastation among projects which had been established to serve or to include young lesbians and gay men. Touring theatre companies were banned, lesbian or gay youth groups had their funding withdrawn, books were removed from council libraries and in one case the Education Officer for East Sussex banned the National Youth Bureau directory of opportunities for volunteers because it contained a single reference to an organisation recruiting lesbian and gay volunteers (Colvin and Hawksley 1989).

Despite official hostility, lesbian and gay youth work has an impressive record of achievement, although, in a climate of vicious homophobia, simply providing a safe space for young lesbians to meet once a week can require months of negotiation and struggle. Yet again, the needs of young lesbians are clearly distinct from those of young gay men. Sexism may impact as much as, if not more than, heterosexism on the lives of young lesbians, and their needs may be more appropriately met within what is known as 'girls' work' than within mixed gay provision. Girls' work originated in the late nineteenth century, when the first youth clubs for girls were set up in the East End of London in response to philanthropic concern about the deprivation experienced by young working-class women (Dixon *et al.* 1989), and by the 1930s the National Association of Girls' Clubs had 325 registered clubs in London alone. With the growing popularity of co-education in the 1940s, separate provision for girls declined and, with the increasing professionalisation of the youth service, women volunteers were largely ousted by trained male workers. Resources which had been established for the use of girls were absorbed into a putatively mixed provision which rapidly became dominated by young men, to the extent that young women were simply pushed out:

[B]y the 1970s young women had all but disappeared from the clubs. After the age of 14 or 15 the needs of girls were not catered for. . . . Workers were concerned primarily with male youth subcultures, male offenders and the problems they presented to society.

(Dixon *et al.* 1989)

It was the growing feminist consciousness of the 'second wave' of the women's movement in the 1970s which provided the spur for a revival of youth service provision aimed at meeting the needs of young women. Lesbian and heterosexual women, working together to establish single-sex provision for girls, were routinely accused of being lesbian and of plotting to convert young women to lesbianism. From the start this made it clear to heterosexual feminists as well as to lesbians that there was a problem with heterosexism as well as sexism, and that the two were related.

Work with young lesbians became an intrinsic part of feminist youth work. Meanwhile, the beginnings of gay youth work had been established, with the setting up in 1976 of the London Gay Teenage Group (LGTG), against establishment hostility (religious organisations such as the Festival of Light were vociferous in condemnation) and with the unpaid labour of youth workers. LGTG had grown out of the Gay Youth Movement (GYM), a scion and eventually a breakaway group of the Campaign for Homosexual Equality (CHE), with the assistance of the Grapevine Sex Education Project in Islington.[5] It is important to recognise that it was solely through the efforts of lesbian and gay youth workers that any kind of lesbian and gay youth service developed. Official bodies such as ILEA, later to take the lead in radical equal opportunities work, were obstructive and antagonistic towards such work in the early stages of its development, and the registration process for LGTG dragged on for over two years.

With the eventual establishment of mixed gay youth provision, it soon became clear that there was a need for separate provision for young lesbians. So, in 1979, the first Young Lesbian Group was established, by lesbians and for lesbians, to be followed through the 1980s by similar groups throughout London. There are groups for Black, Chinese, Cypriot, South Asian, South Armenian and disabled young lesbians, though such initiatives are sparse outside London. Work outside the capital has been slower and more difficult, and provision for young lesbians is still very much confined to major urban areas.

Work with young lesbians is supported by the National Organisation of Lesbian and Gay Youth and Community Workers (NOLGYCW), set up in 1989. NOLGYCW provides trained facilitators who run anti-heterosexism workshops on request, offers support to lesbian and gay workers, lobbies local authorities to provide or to maintain youth service provision for young lesbians and gay men, and, when appropriate, works at a national level. As a voluntary organisation, funded entirely by membership subscription, NOLGYCW is yet another instance of important work being done by lesbian and gay workers concerned about the plight of young lesbians and gays.

Another organisation which is important in terms of work with young lesbians is the National Organisation for Work with Girls and Young Women (NOWGYW), based in Manchester. An umbrella organisation for Young Women's Work, NOWGYW is active in promoting the rights and supporting the needs of young lesbians, whether in mixed (lesbian/ non-lesbian) young women's groups or in lesbian groups. Feminist in ideology and with an analysis which recognises the links between sexism and heterosexism, NOWGYW is particularly sensitive to the needs of young lesbians.

POLICING AND CRIME

Lesbians may be attacked, harassed, victimised and threatened for their sexuality (Comstock 1991, LSPU 1985)[6] and are also vulnerable to sexual assault and rape, yet they receive an inadequate service from the police. The British police appear to be, if anything, more prejudiced than the population in general, and are certainly guilty of maltreatment of lesbian victims of crime (Galloway 1983), though this may be in the process of changing in those connurbations (such as London or Brighton) where lesbian and gay groups have mounted sustained campaigns to raise police awareness of this issue. This is not a problem unique to British society. In his analysis of violence against lesbians and gay men in the USA and Canada, Gary David Comstock comments on 'the frequency of violence by the police' shown up in his own research and substantiated by other sources. He cites the findings of one project in Winnipeg which found:

> [I]n response to calls for assistance by victims of anti-gay/lesbian violence the practice of on-duty police officers is frequently (1) to refuse to intervene, either to protect the victims or to apprehend the prepetrators; (2) to minimise the seriousness of reported incidents, because the victims are lesbian or gay; (3) to blame the victims; and (4) to harass verbally and/or to abuse physically the victims.
>
> (Comstock 1991)

The similarity of this picture to complaints routinely made by British lesbians and gay men about the police is noteworthy. Indeed, so concerned have GALOP/LESPOP[7] become about the abuse of the arrest laws to intimidate lesbians and gay men and the mistreatment of lesbian and gay individuals by the police that they have issued 'bust cards', which give legal advice about police procedures and civil rights for lesbians and gay men who may be arrested.

Although lesbians are less involved than gay men in the production and consumption of pornography and in anonymous public sex (the two areas of most intrusive police interference in the gay community), they are just as likely to be mistreated by police officers when involved in demonstrations, 'zaps' or other public political action, and are more at risk than men from rape and sexual assault. Some anecdotal evidence suggests that lesbians are more unwilling than non-lesbian women to report rape to the police, although there is recent evidence to suggest that, in the area of male violence at least, the police are developing a more sympathetic and appropriate response to lesbian victims of crime (although such evidence is limited to individual experience in regions where for some time the police have been actively monitored and called to acount by the lesbian and gay community).

Since the duty of the police is to enforce the law, and since the law itself directly discriminates against lesbians and gay men, it would be extraordinary if relations between the police and the lesbian and gay communities they serve were anything other than acrimonious. Laws such as Section 28 act amorphously as a legislative justification of homophobia, publicly compromising the right of lesbians to equal and just treatment. In many States of the USA lesbian sexual activity is a criminal offence. Until the law is changed and lesbian and gay citizens are recognised as being entitled to full human and civil rights, there will be little hope, outside those localities where sufficient local pressure can be brought to bear to prompt change, of improving the service offered to lesbians and gay men by the police.

OLDER LESBIANS

The problems visited on elderly women by discriminatory social policy are likely to be exacerbated for lesbian elders. Isolation, poverty and poor housing affect the majority of elderly people in Britain, as else-where in the West, and the majority of those people are women (Pascal 1986). The sexuality of elderly people is denied whatever their sexual orientation, and the needs of older lesbians or gay men are simply not recognised in either the private, charitable or statutory sector (LSPU 1985).[8] Lesbians who are old today will have lived very different lives from those that have been increasingly possible (at least for relatively well-off, urban lesbians) since the 1970s. They have not had access to the social networks and support systems of the contemporary lesbian community and may well have lived and continue to live entirely secret lives. We have no means of knowing how many elderly people are lesbians, but it is likely that many elderly lesbians are living in hardship and loneliness and, given the refusal of the lesbian and gay community to consider the needs of its elders, this is a group likely to remain invisible for some time yet (Neild and Pearson 1992).

LESBIAN HEALTH

There is little recognition within the NHS or other public healthcare systems of the health needs of lesbians. Women make up the bulk of the healthcare workforce, both paid and unpaid. Not only do women comprise over 75 per cent of the NHS workforce (making the NHS the biggest employer of women in Europe) at lower levels and for lower pay than men, but women also provide the vast majority of informal healthcare. Preventing sickness, treating acute illness and injury and caring for the terminally ill and chronically sick or disabled are all activities which take place mostly in the home. A set of activities which occupies so many women for so much time, whether paid or unpaid, must statistically involve large numbers of lesbians, but the needs of lesbian carers and healthcare workers are not recognised by health and social services policies (Royal College of Nursing 1992).

As clients of healthcare, too, the needs of lesbians go unrecognised. Lesbian sexual activity is widely accepted to be much safer than conventional heterosexual activity and, in terms of sexually transmitted diseases such as HIV, chylamidia or gonorrhoea (Hepburn and Gutierrez 1988, O'Donnell *et al.* 1979), lesbians are the lowest-risk sexually active group in the population. Lesbians are, in addition, free from the damaging effects of contraceptive use, and have a less direct relationship to the hazards associated with pregnancy and birth. However, there are health problems which appear to have specific links to lesbian lifestyles. Breast cancer, for example, appears to be statistically more common among lesbians than non-lesbian women (Ross 1992),[9] while drug and alcohol dependency problems are widely accepted to be of major concern in lesbian populations (Faltz 1988, Hepburn and Gutierrez 1988, Pohl 1988). Mental health problems such as anxiety and depression, eating disorders, self-injury and attempted suicide are likely to be influenced by the self-esteem and social support available to lesbians, and research into such issues is just beginning (Ryan and Bradford 1988). In Britain, lesbian healthcare workers are beginning to network.

The need for separate provision for lesbian healthcare is indicated by the experience of the Sandra Bernhardt clinic, an STD clinic catering specifically for lesbians on one afternoon a week at the Charing Cross NHS Hospital in London. Within weeks of opening, demand was so great that the clinic had a six-week waiting list, and lesbians were attending from many NHS regions (Dr Jane Kavanagh 1992, personal communication). There is a new and growing awareness of the needs of this client group. For example, the Royal College of Nursing is currently researching the health care experiences of lesbians and gay men at a national level.

Homophobia is the most obvious concern of lesbians using health-care facilities, whether public or private. Institutional heterosexism – the assumption that heterosexuality is the norm and is innately superior to lesbianism – results in lesbians being ignored as potential users of healthcare facilities. Next-of-kin procedures seldom recognise lesbian partnerships, questions about sexual behaviour or family life assume heterosexuality, and there may be no procedure for dealing with conflict between the family of origin and the family of choice should this arise. Prejudice and misinformation about lesbians among nursing and medical staff is only rarely challenged in their training, and many lesbians who choose to make their sexuality known to hospital or clinic staff report experiencing hostility and poorer-quality care (Dr Jane Kavanagh and Clare Farquahar 1994, personal communication).

Health and healthcare are issues of concern to all lesbians. Yet the history of the medical profession with regard to homosexuality is a troubled and shameful one, ranging from the medical experiments carried out by doctors at Buchenwald, to the widely documented tendency of doctors to reveal their patients' homosexuality to the press. Medical and psychiatric discourse have been instrumental in labelling homosexuality a sickness, and attempts to 'cure' homosexual desire medically have often been brutal. The British Mental Health Act can still be used to detain compulsorily and administer treatment to lesbians or gay men (Armitage *et al.* 1987). In addition, a section of the medical profession has been homophobic in its response to the HIV/AIDS epidemic. A GP in Britain wrote to the British Medical Journal: 'I view homosexuals with the same kind of vague loathing that I view terrorists', while medical students in Moscow declared publicly that AIDS is 'a noble epidemic' ridding society of drug addicts and homosexuals (Watney 1987). It is this history of oppression and abusive treatment at the hands of the medical profession which lesbians carry with them when they seek medical care. Recognition of this fact by heterosexual healthcare professionals is long overdue.

CONCLUSION

Lesbians inhabit a precarious position within the nation-state and are invisible as clients of welfare. In a state which accords citizenship benefits in return for the fulfilment of citizenly duties (to be or to breed fodder for the military machine or the labour force) and which demonises the homosexual as the enemy within, lesbians have a compromised claim to citizenship and stand marked as treacherous. In a society where the heterosexual, nuclear family is naturalised as both healthy and religiously ordained, lesbians stand marked as sick and ungodly. In a state which both assumes and depends on a gendered division of labour there is no place for lesbians.

The major state institutions – education, housing, healthcare and the personal social services – are characterised by ubiquitous heterosexism, sexism and homophobia, putting lesbians in jeopardy on account of both gender and sexuality and refusing to identify and meet the needs of lesbian clients. The law actively discriminates against lesbians, creating a national climate of officially sanctioned homophobia and making it impossible for lesbian citizens to attain a proper and legitimate relationship to the police and courts.

Social policy research, even that which derives from feminist principles, fails almost without exception to examine the effects of social policy on lesbians. Research is urgently needed into many areas affecting lesbians in their relationship to the state. The symbolic function which lesbianism is made to perform in order to maintain the hegemonic order should no longer be allowed to override the civil liberties of lesbian citizens. Providing adequate and appropriate education, healthcare, income maintenance, personal social services and housing for lesbians must be seen not as an aberration or a marginal luxury but as on a par with providing those services for all citizens. And, perhaps most importantly, consensual sexual desire and sexual practice should be redefined as entirely outwith the realm of criminality.

Social policy as an academic discipline fails at its peril to consider lesbians. As with all other areas of study, to neglect the issue of lesbianism warps the perspective which social policy brings to bear on society – without an understanding of the place of lesbianism in social policy it is not possible to fully understand the position of heterosexuality. Additionally, I suggest that it is only within a lesbian-feminist paradigm that the political nature of sexuality and gender as constructs of the contemporary nation-state may be adequately comprehended, and the rights of all citizens guaranteed.

NOTES

1 The Christian church in Britain, certainly, but also the doctrines of Judaism, Islam, Hinduism, Sikhism and other major world religions have been deployed by a male priesthood to ensure women's subordination to the rule of men is reinforced by divine fiat (see Daly 1979, Sahgal and Yuval-Davis 1992). It will be interesting indeed to watch the effect on the Church of England of the Synod's decision (12 November 1992) to allow the ordination of women.

2 A sentiment which noxiously echoes the 'God made Adam and Eve, not Adam and Steve' idiocies of Christian anti-gay rights campaigners in the States!

3 Gay men, of course, although far more likely to be able to afford good-quality housing because of their greater earning power and their social status as men, are currently penalised, when applying for mortgages, by discriminatory practices relating to HIV/AIDS, something not shared by lesbians.

4 'Hidden curriculum' is a phrase used by educationalists to refer to the social learning that takes place informally at schools. Issues such as the relative status of men and women in the school system (canteen staff mostly women, headteachers mostly men, etc.), the representation of male and female characters in textbooks, assumptions about what are appropriate subjects for boy and girl students, careers advice, offering inferior sporting facilities to girl students, all form part of the hidden curriculum as it relates to gender. A similar exercise may be carried out for race, sexuality, class, etc.

5 This excellent and innovative project is now defunct, after the sudden withdrawal of its grant in 1989.

6 It is important to note here that although the extent of domestic violence and sexual violence against women is appalling it is men rather than women (and in particular Black men) who are most at risk from violent assault (Townsend *et al.* 1987). Gay men are 'queerbashed' more frequently than lesbians – violence, like everything else, is 'private' for women and 'public' for men.

7 GALOP is the Gay London Policing project, LESPOP the lesbian equivalent. They are based in London and monitor relations between the lesbian and gay community and the police. It is largely due to their efforts that a handful of senior police officers have made public statements in the last few years indicating their resolve to take anti-gay violence seriously and to promote equality of opportunity for lesbian and gay recruits to the force (see, for example, 'Manchester police chief gives equal opportunities pledge' in *Gay Times*, November 1992).

8 Although a limited amount of private nursing home provision specifically for lesbian and gay elders is available in the USA, this is due to the relative size of the queer population exerting a (small) pressure on the market. This is unlikely to be possible in smaller countries.

9 This may relate to the fact that breast feeding a child appears to offer a significant degree of protection against breast cancer, though alcohol and drug use would also appear to be contributory factors in acquiring the disease.

Bibliography

Jane AARON and Sylvia WALBY (1991) 'Towards a feminist intellectual space', in AARON and WALBY (eds) *Out of the Margins – Women's Studies in the Nineties*, London: Falmer.

Sidney ABBOTT and Barbara LOVE (1972) *Sappho Was a Right-On Woman: a Liberated View of Lesbianism*, New York: Stein and Day.

Pamela ABBOTT and Claire WALLACE (1990) *An Introduction to Sociology: Feminist Perspectives*, London: Routledge.

Parveen ADAMS (1993) 'The three (dis)graces', *New Formations* 19 (Spring), 'Perversity' special issue.

Marcey ADELMAN (1986) *Long Time Passing: Lives of Older Lesbians*, Boston: South End Press.

Peter AGGLETON and Tamsin WILTON (1990) 'AIDS – working with young people', in Peter AGGLETON, Chrissie HORSLEY, Ian WARWICK and Tamsin WILTON, *AIDS – Working with Young People*, Horsham: AVERT.

Margaret ALIC (1986) *Hypatia's Heritage – A History of Women in Science from Antiquity to the Late Nineteenth Century*, London: Women's Press.

Paula Gunn ALLEN (1989) 'Lesbians in American Indian cultures' in DUBERMAN *et al.* (eds) *Hidden from History: Reclaiming the Gay and Lesbian Past*, Harmondsworth, Penguin.

Sue ALLEN and Lyn HARNE (1988) 'Lesbian mothers and the fight for child custody', in Bob CANT and Sue HEMMINGS, *Radical Records – Thirty Years of Lesbian and Gay History*, London: Routledge.

Harriet ALPERT (ed.) (1988) *We Are Everywhere – Writings by and about Lesbian Parents*, Freedom, California: The Crossing Press.

Dennis ALTMAN *et al.* (1989) *Which Homosexuality? Essays from the International Scientific Conference on Lesbian and Gay Studies*, London: Gay Mens's Press.

Sonya ANDERMAHR (1993) 'The worlds of lesbian/feminist science fiction', in Gabriele GRIFFIN (ed.) *Outwrite: Lesbianism and Popular Culture*, London: Pluto Press.

Maya ANGELOU (1971) *Gather Together in My Name*, London: Virago.

B.D. ANTHONY (1982) 'Lesbian client – lesbian therapist: opportunities and challenges in working together', *Journal of Homosexuality* 7: 45–57.

Susan ARDILL and Sue O'SULLIVAN (1987) 'Upsetting an applecart:

difference, desire and lesbian sadomasochism', in Feminist Review Collective (ed.) *Sexuality: A Reader*, London: Virago.

—— (1989) 'Sex in the summer of '88' in *Feminist Review* 31 (Spring).

Gary ARMITAGE, Julienne DICKEY and Sue SHARPLES (1987) *Out of the Gutter: A Survey of the Treatment of Homosexuality by the Press*, London: Campaign for Press and Broadcasting Freedom.

Madeleine ARNOT and Gaby WEINER (eds) (1987) *Gender and the Politics of Schooling*, London: Hutchinson/Open University.

Ti-Grace ATKINSON (1974) *Amazon Odyssey*, New York: Links Books.

Tommi AVICOLLI (1978) 'Images of gays in rock music', in Karla JAY and Allen YOUNG (eds) *Lavender Culture*, New York: Jove/HBJ.

BAD OBJECT CHOICES (eds) (1991) *How Do I Look? Queer Film and Video*, San Francisco: Bay Press.

Josephine BALMER (1984) *Sappho – Poems and Fragments* (translated and introduced), London: Brilliance Books.

Michèle Aina BARALE (1991) 'Below the belt: (un)covering the Well of Loneliness', in Diana Fuss (ed.) *Inside/Out: Lesbian Theories, Gay Theories*, London: Routledge.

Martha Barron BARRETT (1990) *Invisible Lives: The Truth about Millions of Women-Loving Women*, New York: Harper and Row.

Mary BEARD (1931) 'Women at the crossroads', *Independent Woman* 10 (8) August.

Simone de BEAUVOIR (1953) *The Second Sex*, Harmondsworth: Penguin.

Evelyn Torton BECK (ed.) (1982) *Nice Jewish Girls – A Lesbian Anthology*, Boston: Beacon.

Veronica BEECHEY (1978) 'Women and production: a critical analysis of some sociological theories of women's work', in A. KUHN and A.WOLPE (eds) *Feminism and Materialism*, London: Routledge and Kegan Paul.

Paula BENNETT (1992) 'The pea that duty locks: lesbian and feminist hetero-sexual readings of Emily Dickinson's poetry', in Karla JAY and Joanne GLASGOW (eds) *Lesbian Texts and Contexts: Radical Revisions*, London: Onlywomen Press.

Leslie BENNETTS (1993) 'k.d. lang cuts it close', *Vanity Fair*, August.

Marge BERER (1984) *Who Needs Depo Provera?*, London: Community Rights Project.

William BEVERIDGE (1942) *Social Insurance and Allied Services* (The Beveridge Report) London: HMSO.

Lynda BIRKE (1992) 'In pursuit of difference: scientific studies of men and women', in Gill KIRKUP and Laurie SMITH (eds) *Inventing Women: Science, Technology and Gender*, Cambridge: Polity Press.

Inge BLACKMAN and Kathryn PERRY (1990) 'Skirtin the issue: Lesbian fashion for the 1990s', *Feminist Review* 34, Spring: 'Perverse politics: lesbian issues'.

Ruth BLEIER (1991) 'Science and gender: a critique of biology and its theories on women', in Sneja GUNEW (ed.) *A Reader in Feminist Knowledge*, London: Routledge.

Warren J. BLUMENFELD and Diane RAYMOND (1988) *Looking at Gay and Lesbian Life*, Boston: Beacon Press.

Tessa BOFFIN and Jean FRASER (eds) (1991) *Stolen Glances: Lesbians Take Photographs*, London: Pandora.

Sarah BOSTON (1980) *Women Workers and the Trade Unions*, London: Lawrence and Wishart.

John BOSWELL (1991) 'Revolutions, universals and sexual categories', in DUBERMAN *et al.* (eds) *Hidden from History: Reclaiming the Gay and Lesbian Past*, Harmondsworth: Penguin.

Jane BOWERS (1986) 'Women composers in Italy, 1566–1700', in Jane BOWERS and Judith TICK (eds) *Women Making Music: The Western Art Tradition 1150–1950*, Urbana: University of Illinois Press.

Gloria BOWLES and Renate DUELLI-KLEIN (eds)(1983) *Theories of Women's Studies*, London: Routledge and Kegan Paul.

Barbara BRADBY (1993) 'Lesbians and popular music: does it matter who is singing?', in Gabriele GRIFFIN (ed.) *Outwrite: Lesbians in Popular Culture*, London: Pluto.

Marion Zimmer BRADLEY (1982) *The Mists of Avalon*, New York: Ballantine.

Margaret BRADSTOCK and Louise WAKELING (eds) (1987) *Words from the Same Heart*, Sydney: Hale and Ironmonger.

David BRANDON (1981) *Voices of Experience – Consumer Perspectives of Psychiatric Treatment*, London: National Association for Mental Health (MIND).

Philip BRETT, Gary THOMAS and Elizabeth WOOD (eds) (1995) *Queering The Pitch: The New Lesbian and Gay Musicology*, London: Routledge.

Lyndie BRIMSTONE (1991) 'Out of the margins and into the soup: some thoughts on incorporation', in Jane AARON and Sylvia WALBY (eds) *Out of the Margins: Women's Studies in the Nineties*, London: Falmer.

Joseph BRISTOW (ed.) (1992) *Sexual Sameness: Textual Differences in Lesbian and Gay Writing*, London: Routledge.

Nicole BROSSARD (1985) *La Lettre Aerienne*, Montreal: Remue–menage (trans: Marlene Wildeman (1988) *The Aerial Letter*, Toronto: Women's Press).

Judith BROWN (1986) 'Lesbian sexuality in mediaeval and early modern Europe', in *Immodest Acts*, Oxford University Press.

Rita Mae BROWN (1988) 'Historical note on Radicalesbians', in Sarah LUCIA-HOAGLAND and Julia PENELOPE (eds) *For Lesbians Only: A Separatist Anthology*, London: Onlywomen Press.

Beverley BRYAN, Stella DADZIE and Suzanne SCARFE (1987) 'Learning to resist: black women and education', in Gaby WEINER and Madeleine ARNOT (eds) *Gender under Scrutiny*, Milton Keynes: Open University Press.

Elly BULKIN (1981) 'Lesbian short fiction in the classroom', in *Lesbian Fiction: An Anthology*, Watertown, Mass: Persephone Press.

Paul BURSTON (1992) 'The death of queer politics', in *Gay Times*, August.

Becky BUTLER (ed.) (1990) *Ceremonies of the Heart: Celebrating Lesbian Unions*, Seal Press.

Judith BUTLER (1990) *Gender Trouble: Feminism and the Subversion of Identity*, London: Routledge.

—— (1993) 'Critically queer', *GLQ: A Journal of Lesbian and Gay Studies* 1(1): 17–32.

Mary S. CALDERONE and Eric W. JOHNSON (1989) *The Family Book about Sexuality*, New York: Harper and Row.

Pat CALIFIA (1988) *Sapphistry: The Book of Lesbian Sexuality*, Tallahassee, Florida: Naiad Press.

—— (1991) *The Advocate Adviser*, Boston: Alyson.

—— (1993) 'Sex and Madonna, or, what did you expect from a girl who doesn't put out on the first five dates?', in Lisa FRANK and Paul SMITH (eds) *Madonnarama: Essays on Sex and Popular Culture*, Pittsburgh: Cleis Press.

CAMERAWORK and The Photo Co-op (1989) *Bodies of Experience: Stories about Living with HIV* (exhibition catalogue), London.

Bea CAMPBELL (1980) 'A feminist sexual politics: now you see it, now you don't', *Feminist Review* 5: 1–18.

Bob CANT and Susan HEMMNGS (eds) (1988) *Radical Records – Thirty Years of Lesbian and Gay History*, London: Routledge.

Frank CAPRIO (1957) *Female Homosexuality*, London: Peter Owen.

Claudia CARD (ed.) (1992) 'Lesbian Philosophy', *Hypatia: A Journal of Feminist Philosophy* 7(4).

Terry CASTLE (1992) 'Sylvia Townsend Warner and the counterplot of lesbian fiction', in Joseph BRISTOW (ed.) *Sexual Sameness: Textual Differences in Lesbian and Gay Writing*, London: Routledge.

Whitney CHADWICK (1990) *Women, Art and Society*, London: Thames and Hudson.

CHAR (Housing Campaign for Single People) (1988) *Housing for Lesbians and Gay Men* (report of a conference held on 1 October).

Helen (charles) 'Whiteness – the relevance of politically colouring the "non"', in Hilary HINDS, Ann PHOENIX and Jackie STACEY (eds) *Working Out: New Directions for Women's Studies*, London: Falmer.

Nickie CHARLES (1993) *Gender Divisions and Social Change*, London: Harvester Wheatsheaf.

Nicola CHARLES (1986) 'Women and trade unions', in Feminist Review Collective (eds) *Waged Work: A Reader*, London: Virago.

Kate CHARLESWORTH (1984) *Exotic Species: A Field Guide to Some of our British Gays*, London: Gay Men's Press.

George CHAUNCEY Jnr., Martin DUBERMAN and Martha VICINUS (1989) 'Introduction', in *Hidden From History: Reclaiming the Gay and Lesbian Past*, Harmondsworth: Penguin.

J.W. CHESEBRO (1981) 'Introduction', in CHESEBRO (ed.) *Gayspeak*, New York: Pilgrim Press.

Judy CHICAGO (1979) *The Dinner Party: A Symbol of Our Heritage*, New York: Anchor/Doubleday.

—— (1980) *Embroidering Our Heritage: The Dinner Party Needlework*, New York: Anchor/Doubleday.

Sarah CHINN and Kris FRANKLIN (1992) '"I am what I am" (or am I?): the making and unmaking of lesbian and gay identity in *High Tech Gays*,' in Cheryl KADER and Thomas PIONTEK (eds) *Discourse* 15(1) Fall: 'Essays in Lesbian and Gay Studies'.

Carol P. CHRIST (1991) 'Why women need the goddess: phenomenological and psychological reflections', in Sneja GUNEW, *A Reader in Feminist Knowledge*, London: Routledge.

Debbie CLARKE (1988) 'Equal opportunities for all? Lesbians and health care', in *Radical Community Medicine*, Winter.

Wendy CLARKE (1982) 'The dyke, the feminist and the devil', *Feminist Review* 11: 30–9.

Katherine CLARRICOATES (1987) 'Dinosaurs in the classroom – the "hidden" curriculum in primary schools', in Madeleine ARNOT and Gaby WEINER (eds) *Gender and the Politics of Schooling*, Milton Keynes: Open University Press.
CLIT COLLECTIVE (1974) 'C.L.I.T. Statement No. 2' reprinted in Sarah LUCIA-HOAGLAND and Julia PENELOPE (eds) (1988) *For Lesbians Only: A Separatist Anthology*, London: Onlywomen Press.
Cynthia COCKBURN (1987) *Women, Trade Unions and Political Parties*, Fabian Research Series 349: London.
—— (1987) *Two-Track Training: Sex Inequalities in the YTS*, London: Macmillan.
—— (1991) *Brothers: Male Dominance and Technological Change*, London: Pluto Press.
Diana COLLECOTT (1992) 'A study in textual inversion', in Joseph BRISTOW (ed.) *Sexual Sameness: Textual Differences in Lesbian and Gay Writing*, London: Routledge.
Patricia Hill COLLINS (1990) *Black Feminist Thought*, London: Harper Collins.
Rose COLLIS (1992) 'Taking it's toll', *Gay Times*, November.
—— (1992) 'Excursions into lesbian erotica', *Gay Times*, January: 40–3.
Madaleine COLVIN and Jane HAWKSLEY (1989) *Section 28: A Practical Guide to The Law and its Implications*, London: Liberty.
COMBAHEE RIVER COLLECTIVE (1982) 'A Black feminist statement', in Glora T. HULL, Patricia Bell SCOTT and Barbara SMITH (eds) *All The Women Are White, All The Black Are Men, But Some Of Us Are Brave: Black Women's Studies*, Old Westbury, NY: The Feminist Press.
Gary David COMSTOCK (1991) *Violence Against Lesbians and Gay Men*, New York: Columbia University Press.
Steve CONNOR and Martin WHITFIELD (1993) 'Scientists at odds in "gay gene" debate', The *Guardian* 17 July: 3.
Juliet COOK and Shantu WATT (1993) 'Racism, women and poverty', in Caroline GLENDINNING and Jane MILLAR (eds) *Women and Poverty in Britain: The 1990s*, London: Harvester Wheatsheaf.
Davina COOPER (1989) 'Positive images in Harringey: a struggle for identity', in Carol JONES and Pat MAHONY (eds) *Learning Our Lines: Sexuality and Social Control in Education*, London: Women's Press.
Anna COOTE and Beatrix CAMPBELL (1987) *Sweet Freedom*, Oxford: Basil Blackwell.
Anna COOTE and Polly PATTULLO (1990) *Power and Prejudice: Women and Politics*, London: Weidenfeld and Nicholson.
Jeanne CORDOVA (1992) 'Butches, lies and feminism', in Joan NESTLE (ed.) *The Persistent Desire: A Femme-Butch Reader*, Boston: Alyson.
Gena COREA (1985) *The Mother Machine: Reproductive Technologies from Artificial Insemination to Artificial Wombs*, London: The Women's Press.
Donald COREY (1965) *Lesbianism in America*, New York: MacFadden.
Paul CRANE (1982) *Gays and The Law*, London: Pluto Press.
Mary CRAWFORD (1993) 'Identity, "passing" and subversion', in Sue WILKINSON and Celia KITZINGER (eds) *Heterosexuality: A Feminism and Psychology Reader*, London: Sage.
Douglas CRIMP with Adam ROLSTON (1990) *AIDS Demo/Graphics*, Seattle: Bay Press.

Margaret CRUIKSHANK (1982) *Lesbian Studies: Present and Future*, New York: The Feminist Press.

—— (ed.) (1985) *The Lesbian Path*, San Francisco: Grey Fox Press.

—— (1992) *The Gay and Lesbian Liberation Movement*, London: Routledge.

Rosemary CURB and Nancy MANAHAN (eds) (1985) *Lesbian Nuns: Breaking Silence*, Tallahassee, Florida, Naiad Press.

Mary DALY (1979) *Gyn/Ecology: The Metaethics of Radical Feminism*, London: The Women's Press.

—— (1984) *Pure Lust: Elemental Feminist Philosophy*, London: The Women's Press.

Mary DALY and Jane CAPUTI (1988) *Wickedary*, London: The Women's Press.

Robert DANIEL and Mark BRILL (1991) 'Children of the rave-olution', *Rouge* 7 (July–September).

Trudy DARTY and Sandee POTTER (1984) *Women-Identified Women*, Paolo Alto: Mayfield.

Neil DAVIDSON (1990) *Boys Will Be . . .? Sex Education and Young Men*, London: Bedford Square Press.

Angela DAVIS (1982) *Women, Race and Class*, London: The Women's Press.

Amy DEAN with Linda WELLS and Andrea CURRAN (1989) *Cut-Outs and Cut-Ups: A Lesbian Fun'n'Games Book*, Norwich, Vermont: New Victoria.

DELORES (1993) 'Phranc' (interview), *LIP* 1.

DEPARTMENT OF HEALTH AND SOCIAL SECURITY (1982) *Supplementary Benefits Handbook*, London.

Rhonda DICKSION (1990) *The Lesbian Survival Manual*, Tallahassee, Florida: Naiad Press.

DIVERSION (1991) *Nottingham and East Midlands Lesbian Magazine* (no date, no artist credit).

Jane DIXON, Gilly SALVAT and Jane SKEATES (1989) 'North London Young Lesbian Group: specialist work within the youth service', in Carol JONES and Pat MAHONY (eds) *Learning Our Lines: Sexuality and Social Control in Education*, London: The Women's Press.

Jonathan DOLLIMORE (1991) *Sexual Dissidence: Augustine to Wilde, Freud to Foucault*, Oxford: Oxford University Press.

DOLORES (1991) 'Skirting the issue? Or well-suited women', *The Pink Paper* 205, 14 December.

Emma DONOGHUE (1993) *Passions Between Women: British Lesbian Culture 1669–1801*, London: Scarlet Press.

Carol Anne DOUGLAS (1990) *Love and Politics: Radical Feminist and Lesbian Theories*, San Francisco: ism press.

Lesley DOYAL (1995) *What Makes Women Sick? Gender and the Political Economy of Health*, London: Macmillan.

Lesley DOYAL with Imogen PENNELL (1979) *The Political Economy of Health*, London: Pluto Press.

Lesley DOYAL and Mary Ann ELSTON (1986) 'Women, health and medicine', in Veronic BEECHEY and Elizabeth WHITELEGG (eds) *Women in Britain Today*, Milton Keynes: Open University Press.

Martin Bauml DUBERMAN, Martha VICINUS, George CHAUNCEY Jnr. (eds) (1991) *Hidden from History: Reclaiming the Gay and Lesbian Past*, Harmondsworth, Penguin.

N. Leigh DUNLAP (1987) *Morgan Calabrese: The Movie*, Norwich, Vermont: New Victoria.

—— (1989) *Run That Sucker at Six*, Norwich, Vermont: New Victoria.

Gill DUNNE (1992) 'Difference at work: perceptions of work from a non-heterosexual perspective', in Hilary HINDS, Ann PHONIX and Jackie STACEY (eds) *Working Out: New Directions for Women's Studies*, London: Falmer Press.

Andrea DWORKIN (1977) 'Biological superiority: the world's most dangerous and deadly idea', in DWORKIN (1988) *Letters from a War Zone: Writings 1976–1987*, London: Secker and Warburg.

—— (1987) *Intercourse*, London: Arrow.

Richard DYER (1990) *Now You See It: Studies on Lesbian and Gay Film*, London: Routledge.

Muriel DYMEN (1984) 'Politically correct? Politically incorrect?', in Carol VANCE (ed.) *Pleasure and Danger: Exploring Female Sexuality*, London: Pandora.

Tim EDWARDS (1994) *Erotics and Politics: Gay Male Sexuality, Masculinity and Feminism*, London: Routledge.

Barbara EHRENREICH and Dierdre ENGLISH (1973) *Complaints and Disorders: The Sexual Politics of Sickness*, London: Writers and Readers Publishing Co-operative.

—— (1979) *For Her Own Good: 150 Years of the Experts' Advice to Women*, London: Pluto.

Anne EISENBERG (1991) 'Quantum English', *Scientific American*, October: 110.

John d'EMILIO (1983) *Sexual Politics, Sexual Communities – the Making of a Homosexual Minority in the United States 1940–1970*, Chicago: University of Chicago Press.

John d'EMILIO and Estelle B. FREEDMAN (1988) *Intimate Matters: A History of Sexuality in America*, New York: Harper and Row.

Julia EPSTEIN and Kristina STRAUB (eds) (1991) *Body Guards: The Cultural Politics of Gender Ambiguity*, London: Routledge.

Steven EPSTEIN (1990) 'Gay politics, ethnic identity: the limits of social constructionism', in Edward STEIN (ed.) *Forms of Desire: Sexual Orientation and the Social Constructionist Controversy*, London: Routledge.

EQUAL OPPORTUNITIES COMMISSION (EOC) (1982a) *Caring for the Elderly and Handicapped: Community Care Policies and Women's Lives*, Manchester.

EOC (1982b) *Who Cares for the Carers? Opportunities for those Caring for the Elderly and Handicapped*, Manchester.

EOC (1984) *Carers and Services: A Comparison of Men and Women Caring for Dependent Elderly People*, Manchester.

Lillian FADERMAN (1981) *Surpassing the Love of Men: Romantic Friendships and Love Between Women from the Renaissance to the Present*, London: The Women's Press.

—— (1991) *Odd Girls and Twilight Lovers: A History of Lesbian Life in Twentieth Century America*, Harmondsworth: Penguin.

Barbara FALZ (1988) 'Substance abuse and the lesbian and gay community assessment and intervention', in Michael SHORNOFF and William STOTT (eds) *The Sourcebook of Lesbian/Gay Healthcare*, Washington: Nation Lesbian and Gay Health Foundation.

Annabel FARADAY (1981) 'Liberating lesbian research', in Ken PLUMMER (ed.) *The Making of the Modern Homosexual*, London: Hutchinson.

Marilyn FARWELL (1992) 'Heterosexual plots and lesbian subtexts', in Karla JAY and Joanne GLASGOW (eds) *Lesbian Texts and Contexts: Radical Revisions*, London: Onlywomen Press.

Feminist Review Collective (eds) (1986) *Waged Work: A Reader*, London: Virago.

Nicola FIELD (1991) 'The moon is shining bright as day – parents, children and Section 28', in Tara KAUFMANN and Paul LINCOLN (eds) *High Risk Lives: Lesbian and Gay Politics after THE CLAUSE*, Bridport: Prism Press.

Rachel FIELD (1990) 'Lesbian tradition', *Feminist Review* 34, Spring: 'Perverse politics: lesbian issues'.

Shulamith FIRESTONE (1970) *The Dialectic of Sex: The Case for Female Revolution*, London: The Women's Press.

Andrea FISHER (1987) *Let Us Now Praise Famous Women: Women Photographers for the US Government 1935 to 1944*, London: Pandora.

Sabina FLANAGAN (1989) *Hildegard of Bingen: A Visionary Life*, London: Routledge.

Margaret FORSTER (1993) *Daphne du Maurier*, London: Chatto and Windus.

Olivia FOSTER-CARTER (1987) 'Racial bias in children's literature' in Gaby WEINER and Madeleine ARNOT (eds) *Gender Under Scrutiny*, Milton Keynes: Open University Press.

Michel FOUCAULT (1976, trans. 1979) *The History of Sexuality Vol. 1: An Introduction*, Harmondsworth: Penguin.

Lisa FRANK and Paul SMITH (eds) (1993) *Madonnarama: Essays on Sex and Popular Culture*, San Francisco: Cleis Press.

Sarah FRANKLIN and Jackie STACEY (1986) *Lesbian Perspectives on Women's Studies*, University of Kent at Canterbury: Women's Studies Occasional Papers.

Estelle FREEDMAN, Barbara GELPI, Susan JOHNSON and Kathleen WESTON (1984) 'Editorial', *Signs* 9(4) Summer.

—— (1985) 'Introduction', *The Lesbian Issue: Essays from "Signs"*, Chicago: University of Chicago Press.

Sigmund FREUD (1905) 'Three essays on the theory of sexuality', in James STRACHEY (ed. and trans.) *Standard Edition of the Complete Psychological Works*, 7: 125–246, London: Hogarth Press.

Richard FUNG (1991) 'Looking for my penis: The eroticized Asian in gay video porn', in BAD OBJECT-CHOICES (eds) *How do I Look? Queer Film and Video*, Seattle: Bay Press.

Diana FUSS (1989) *Essentially Speaking: Feminism, Nature and Difference*, London: Routledge.

—— (1991) 'Inside/out' in FUSS (ed.) *Inside/Out: Lesbian Theories, Gay Theories*, London: Routledge.

Bruce GALLOWAY (ed.) (1983) *Prejudice and Pride: Discrimination against Gay People in Britain*, London: Routledge and Kegan Paul.

Ann GAME (1991) *Undoing the Social: Towards a Deconstructive Sociology*, Milton Keynes: Open University Press.

Marjorie GARBER (1992) *Vested Interests: Cross-Dressing and Cultural Anxiety*, London: Routledge.

Mary GARRARD (1976) 'Of men, women and art: some historical reflections', *Art Journal* xxviv, Summer.

Moira GATENS (1991) 'A critique of the sex/gender distinction', in Sneja GUNEW (ed.) *A Reader in Feminist Knowledge*, London: Routledge.

GAY TEACHERS' GROUP (1987) *School's Out: Lesbian and Gay Rights in Education*, London.

Sally GEARHEART (1974) *Loving Women*, Boston: Alyson.

Anthony GIDDENS (1989) *Sociology*, Cambridge: Polity Press.

—— (1992) *The Transformation of Intimacy*, London: Polity Press.

Charlotte Perkins GILMAN (1911) *The Man-Made Word or Our Androcentric Culture*, London: T. Fisher Unwin.

Joanne GLASGOW (1992) 'What's a nice lesbian like you doing in the Church of Torquemada? Radclyffe Hall and Other Catholic Converts', in Karla JAY and Joanne GLASGOW (eds) *Lesbian Texts and Contexts: Radical Revisions*, London: Onlywomen Press.

Erick GOODE and Richard TROIDEN (eds) (1974) *Sexual Deviance and Sexual Deviants*, New York: Morrow.

Lizbeth GOODMAN (1993) *Feminist Theatres: To Each Her Own*, London: Routledge.

Linda GORDON (1991) 'What's new in women's history', in Sneja GUNEW (ed.) *A Reader in Feminist Knowledge*, London: Routledge.

Della GRACE (1991) *Love Bites*, London: Gay Men's Press.

—— (1993) 'Xenomorphosis', *New Formations* 19, Spring: 'Perversity'.

Hilary GRAHAM (1993) 'Budgeting for health: mothers in low-income households' in Caroline GLENDINNING and Jane MILLAR (eds) *Women and Poverty in Britain: The 1990s*, London, Harvester–Wheatsheaf.

Judy GRAHN (1983) 'Edward the Dyke and other poems', in Stephen COOTE (ed.) *The Penguin Book of Homosexual Verse*, Harmondsworth, Penguin.

—— (1984) *Another Mother Tongue: Gay Words, Gay Worlds*, Boston: Beacon Press.

—— (1985) 'A heart-shaped journey to a similar place', in *The Highest Apple*, San Francisco: Spinsters Ink.

GREATER LONDON COUNCIL and GLC GAY WORKING PARTY (1985) *Changing the World – A London Charter for Gay and Lesbian Rights*, London Strategic Policy Unit.

Dorsey GREEN and Frederick BOZETT (1991) 'Lesbian mothers and gay fathers', in John GONSIOREK and James WEINRICH (eds) *Homosexuality: Research Implications for Public Policy*, London: Sage.

René GREMAUX (1989) 'Mannish women of the Balkan Mountains: preliminary notes', in Jan BREMMER (ed.) *From Sappho to de Sade: Moments in the History of Sexuality*, London: Routledge.

Germaine GREER (1970a) 'The politics of female sexuality' (from 'Cunt Power' issue of *Oz*) reprinted in GREER (1986) *The Madwoman's Underclothes*, New York: Atlantic Monthly Press.

—— (1971) *The Female Eunuch*, London: Granada.

—— (1979) *The Obstacle Race: The Fortunes of Women Painters and Their Work*, London: Secker and Warburg.

Christine GRIFFIN (1987) 'Young women and the transition from school to un/employment: a cultural analysis', in Gaby WEINER and Madeleine ARNOT (eds) *Gender under Scrutiny*, Milton Keynes: Open University Press.

Gabrielle GRIFFIN (ed.) (1993) *Outwrite: Lesbianism and Popular Culture*, London: Pluto Press.

Elizabeth GROSS (1992) 'What is feminist theory?', in Helen CROWLEY and Susan HIMMELWEIT, *Knowing Women – Feminism and Knowledge*, Cambridge: Polity Press.

Elizabeth GROSZ (1990a) 'Conclusion: a note on essentialism and difference', in Sneja GUNEW (ed.) *Feminist Knowledge: Critique and Construct*, London: Routledge.

—— (1990b) 'Contemporary theories of power and subjectivity', in Sneja GUNEW (ed.) *Feminist Knowledge: Critique and Construct*, London: Routledge.

Ian HACKING (1990) 'Making up people', in Edward STEIN (ed.) *Forms of Desire: Sexual Orientation and the Social Constructionist Controversy*, London: Routledge.

Erwin J. HAEBERLE (1981) '"Stigmata of degeneration": prisoner markings in Nazi concentration camps', in Salvatore LICATA and Robert PETERSEN (eds) *Historical Perspectives on Homosexuality*, New York: The Haworth Press.

—— (1989) 'Swastika, pink triangle and yellow star: the destruction of sexology and the persecution of homosexuals in Nazi Germany', in Martin Bauml DUBERMAN *et al.* (eds) (1991) *Hidden from History: Reclaiming the Gay and Lesbian Past*, Harmondsworth: Penguin.

Dorothy HAGE (1972) 'There's glory for you', in *Aphra: The Feminist Literary Magazine* 3(3): 2–14.

Gill HAGUE and Ellen MALOS (1993) *Domestic Violence: Action for Change*, Cheltenham: New Clarion Press.

Jacquelyn Dowd HALL (1984) 'The mind that burns in each body: women, rape and racial violence', in Anne SNITOW *et al.* (eds) *Desire: The Politics of Sexuality*, London: Virago.

HALL CARPENTER ARCHIVES LESBIAN ORAL HISTORY GROUP (1989) *Inventing Ourselves: Lesbian Life Stories*, London: Routledge.

David HALPERIN (1991) 'Sex before sexuality: pederasty, politics and power in Classical Athens', in Martin Bauml DUBERMAN *et al.* (eds) *Hidden from History: Reclaiming the Gay and Lesbian Past*, Harmondsworth: Penguin.

Christopher HAM (1992) *Health Policy in Britain*, London: Macmillan.

Diane HAMER and Belinda BUDGE (eds) (1994) *The Good, The Bad and The Gorgeous: Lesbianism and Popular Culture*, London: Scarlet Press.

Diane HAMER, Paul LINCOLN and Tara KAUFMANN (1991) 'Lifestyle or practice? A new target for legislation', in KAUFMANN *et al.* (eds) *High Risk Lives: Lesbian and Gay Politics after THE CLAUSE*, Bridport: Prism Press.

June HANNAM (1993) 'Women, history and protest', in Diane RICHARDSON and Victoria ROBINSON (eds) *Introducing Women's Studies*, London: Macmillan.

Karen HARBECK (1992) 'Introduction' in HARBECK (ed.) *Coming Out of the Classroom Closet: Gay and Lesbian Students, Teachers and Curricula*, New York: Harrington Park Press.

Simon HARRIS (1990) *Lesbian and Gay Issues in the English Classroom*, Milton Keynes: Open University Press.

John HART and Diane RICHARDSON (eds) (1981) *The Theory and Practice of Homosexuality*, London: Routledge and Kegan Paul.

HARVARD LAW REVIEW (eds) (1989) *Sexual Orientation and The Law*, Cambridge, Mass: Harvard University Press.

Rachel HASTED (1989) 'Queen for a night', *Trouble and Strife* 17: 32–8.

Susan HAWTHORNE (1991) 'In Defence of separatism', in Sneja GUNEW (ed.) *A Reader in Feminist Knowledge*, London: Routledge.

Kirsten HEARN (1988) 'Oi! What about us?' in Bob CANT and Susan HEMMINGS (eds) *Radical Records: Thirty Years of Lesbian and Gay History*, London: Routledge.

—— (1991) 'Disabled lesbians and gays are here to stay!', in Tara KAUFMANN and Paul LINCOLN (eds) *High Risk Lives: Lesbian and Gay Politics after THE CLAUSE*, Bridport: Prism Press.

Nancy G. HELLER (1987) *Women Artists: An Illustrated History*, London: Abbeville Press.

Susan HEMMINGS (1986) 'Overdose of doctors', in Sue O'SULLIVAN (ed.) (1987) *Women's Health: A Spare Rib Reader*, London: Pandora.

Alison HENNEGAN (1988) 'On becoming a lesbian reader', in Susannah RADSTONE (ed.) *Sweet Dreams: Sexuality, Gender and Popular Fiction*, London: Lawrence and Wishart.

Cuca HEPBURN with Bonnie GUTIERREZ (1988) *Alive and Well: A Lesbian Health Guide*, Freedom, California: The Crossing Press.

Gilbert HERDT (ed.) (1989) *Gay and Lesbian Youth*, New York: The Haworth Press.

Gregory HEREK (1991) 'Stigma, prejudice and violence against lesbians and gay men', in John GONSIOREK and James WEINRICH (eds) *Homosexuality: Research Implications for Public Policy*, London: Sage.

HETRICK-MARTIN INSTITUTE (1988) *Tales of the Closet* 1(3): 'Violence', New York.

—— (1989) *Tales of the Closet* 1(4): 'Health', New York.

David HEVEY (1992) *The Creatures Time Forgot: Photography and Disability Imagery*, London: Routledge.

Elaine HOBBY and Chris WHITE (eds) (1991) *What Lesbians Do in Bed*, London: The Women's Press.

Barbara Meil HOBSON (1987) *Uneasy Virtue: The Politics of Prostitution and the American Reform Tradition*, New York: Bantam Books.

Amber HOLLIBAUGH and Cherríe MORAGA (1984) 'What we're rolling around in bed with: sexual silences in feminism', in Ann SNITOW *et al.* (eds) *Desire: The Politics of Sexuality*, London: Virago.

Sarah HOLMES (ed.) (1988) *Testimonies: A Collection of Lesbian Coming Out Stories*, Boston: Alyson.

Hilary HOMANS (ed.) (1985) *The Sexual Politics of Reproduction*, Aldershot: Gower.

bell hooks (1990) 'The politics of radical black subjectivity', in *Yearning: Race, Gender and Cultural Politics*, Boston: South End Press.

Valentine HOOVEN III (1992) *Tom of Finland (Introduction)*, Koln: Benedict Taschen Verlag.

Nym HUGHES, Yvonne JOHNSON and Yvete PERRAULT (1984) *Stepping Out of Line: A Workbook on Lesbianism and Feminism*, Vancouver: Press Gang.

Laud HUMPHREYS (1970) *The Tearoom Trade*, London: Duckworth.

Margaret HUNT (1981) 'Report of a conference on feminism, sexuality and power: the elect clash with the perverse', in SAMOIS (eds) *Coming to Power: Writings and Graphics on Lesbian S/M*, Boston: Alyson.

—— (1990) 'The de-eroticization of women's liberation: social purity movements and the revolutionary feminism of Sheila Jeffreys', in *Feminist Review* 34: 'Perverse politics: lesbian issue'.

Marsha HUNT (1990) *Joy: A novel*, London: Century Hutchinson.

Richard A. ISAY (1989) *Being Homosexual: Gay Men and Their Development*, Harmondsworth: Penguin.

Joanne ISSACK (1985) 'Women: the ruin of representation', *Afterimage* 12(9): 3–11.

Cath JACKSON (1984) *Wonder Wimbin: Everyday Stories of Feminist Folk*, London: Battle Axe Books.

—— (1986) *Visibly Vera*, London: The Women's Press.

Gabriel JAFFE (1961) *The Life Pill*, London: Consul Books.

Derek JARMAN (1991) *Queer Edward II*, London: British Film Institute.

Karla JAY and Joanne GLASGOW (eds) (1992) *Lesbian Texts and Contexts: Radical Revisions*, London: Onlywomen Press.

Sheila JEFFREYS (1985) *The Spinster and Her Enemies: Feminism and Sexuality 1880–1930*, London: Pandora.

—— (1989) 'Does it matter if they did it?', in LESBIAN HISTORY GROUP *Not a Passing Phase: Reclaiming Lesbians in History 1840–1985*, London: The Women's Press.

—— (1990) *Anticlimax: A Feminist Perspective on the Sexual Revolution*, London: The Women's Press.

Carol JONES and Pat MAHONY (eds) (1989) *Learning Our Lines: Sexuality and Social Control in Education*, London: The Women's Press.

Nicholas de JONGH (1992) *Not in Front of the Audience: Homosexuality on Stage*, London: Routledge.

Cheryl KADER and Thomas PIONTEK (eds) (1992) *Discourse: Theoretical Studies in Media and Culture* 15(1) (Fall): 'Essays in lesbian and gay studies'.

Kadiatu KANNEH (1993) 'Sisters under the skin: a politics of heterosexuality', in Sue WILKINSON and Celia KITZINGER (eds) *Heterosexuality: A Feminism and Psychology Reader*, London: Sage.

Gisela KAPLAN and Lesley ROGERS (1991) 'The definition of male and female: biological reductionism and the sanctions of normality', in Sneja GUNEW (ed.) *Feminist Knowledge: Critique and Construct*, London: Routledge.

Mumtaz KARIMJEE (1991) 'In search of an image', *Trouble and Strife* 20, Spring.

Jonathan Ned KATZ (1983) *Gay/Lesbian Alamanac: A New Documentary*, New York: Harper and Row.

Tara KAUFMANN and Paul LINCOLN (eds) (1991) *High Risk Lives: Lesbian and Gay Politics after THE CLAUSE*, Bridport: Prism Press.

Alison KELLY (1987) 'The construction of masculine science', in Madeleine

ARNOT and Gaby WEINER (eds) *Gender and the Politics of Schooling*, London: Hutchinson/Open University.

Liz KELLY, Linda REGAN and Sheila BURTON (1992) 'Defending the indefensible? Quantitative methods and feminist research', in Hilary HINDS, Ann PHOENIX and Jackie STACEY (eds) *Working Out: New Directions for Women's Studies*, London: Falmer.

Sandra KESSLER, Dean ASHENDEN, Bob CONNELL and Gary DOWSETT (1987) 'Gender relations in secondary schooling', in ARNOT and WEINER (eds) *Gender and the Politics of Schooling*, London: Hutchinson/Open University.

KILLA-MAN (1974) 'Trying hard to forfeit all I've known', in Sarah LUCIA-HOAGLAND and Julia PENELOPE (eds) (1988) *For Lesbians Only: A Separatist Anthology*, London: Onlywomen Press.

Katie KING (1990) 'Producing sex, theory and culture: gay/straights remappings in contemporary feminism', in Marianne HIRSCH and Evelyn FOX-KELLER (eds) *Conflicts in Feminism*, London: Routledge.

KISS AND TELL (1991) *Drawing the Line: Lesbian Sexual Politics on the Wall*, Vancouver: Press Gang.

Celia KITZINGER (1987) *The Social Construction of Lesbianism*, London: Sage.

—— (1990) 'Heterosexism in psychology', *The Psychologist*, September.

—— (1991) 'Politicizing psychology', *Feminism and Psychology* 1(1) London: Sage.

Celia KITZINGER, Sue WILKINSON and Rachel PERKINS (1993) 'Theorizing heterosexuality', in Sue WILKINSON and Celia KITZINGER (eds) *Heterosexuality: A Feminism and Psychology Reader*, London: Sage.

Celia KITZINGER and Rachel PERKINS (1993) *Changing Our Minds*, London: Onlywomen Press.

Dolores KLAICH (1985) *Woman Plus Woman*, Tallahassee, Naiad Press.

Wayne KOESTENBAUM (1991) 'The queen's throat: (Homo)sexuality and the art of singing', in Diana FUSS (ed.) *Inside/Out: Lesbian Theories, Gay Theories*, London: Routledge.

Heinrich KRAMER and James SPRENGER (1486 trans. 1946, ed. 1971) *Malleus Maleficarum*, London: Arrow.

Cheris KRAMERAE and Paula TREICHLER (1985) *A Feminist Dictionary*, London: Pandora.

Annette KUHN (1988) *Cinema, Censorship and Sexuality 1909–1925*, London: Routledge.

Sandra LAHIRE (1987) 'Lesbians in media education', in Hilary ROBINSON (ed.) *Visibly Female: Feminism and Art Today*, London: Camden Press.

Rita LAPORTE (1976) 'Sex and sexuality', in Barbara GRIER and Colette REID (eds) *The Lavender Herring: Lesbian Essays from The Ladder*, Baltimore: Diana Press.

Robert LAPSLEY and Michael WESTLAKE (1988) *Film Theory: An Introduction*, Manchester University Press.

André LARDINOIS (1989) 'Lesbian Sappho and the Sappho of Lesbos', in Jan Bremmer (ed.) *From Sappho to De Sade: Moments in the History of Sexuality*, London: Routledge.

Teresa de LAURETIS (1991) 'Film and the visible', in BAD OBJECT-

CHOICES (eds) *How Do I Look? Queer Film and Video*, San Francisco: Bay Press.

Sophie LAWS, Valerie HEY and Andrea EAGAN (1985) *Seeing Red: The Politics of Pre-Menstrual Tension*, London: Hutchinson.

LEEDS REVOLUTIONARY FEMINIST GROUP (1981) 'Political lesbianism: the case against heterosexuality', in *Love Your Enemy*, London: Onlywomen Press.

Zoë LEONARD (1990) 'Lesbians in the AIDS Crisis' in ACT UP/NEW YORK WOMEN AND AIDS BOOK GROUP (eds) *Women, AIDS and Activism*, Boston: South End Press.

LESBIAN HISTORY GROUP (1989) *Not a Passing Phase: Reclaiming Lesbians in History 1840–1985*, London: The Women's Press.

Anna LIVIA (ed. and trans.) (1993) *A Perilous Advantage: the Best of Natalie Clifford Barney*, New Victoria Publishers.

LONDON STRATEGIC POLICY UNIT (1985) *Changing the World: A London Charter for Gay and Lesbian Rights*, London: GLC.

Audre LORDE (1979) 'The Master's tools will never dismantle the master's house', in Andre LORDE (1984) *Sister Outsider: Essays and Speeches*, Trumansberg NY: The Crossing Press.

—— (1982) *Zami: A New Spelling of My Name*, London: Sheba.

JoAnn LOULAN (1987) *Lesbian Passion: Loving Ourselves and Each Other*, San Francisco: Spinsters/ Aunt Lute.

Marian LOWE and Margaret LOWE BENSTON (1991) 'The uneasy alliance of feminism and academia', in Sneja GUNEW (ed.) *A Reader in Feminist Knowledge*, London: Routledge.

Sarah LUCIA-HOAGLAND (1988) *Lesbian Ethics: Towards New Value*, Palo Alto, California: Institute of Lesbian Studies.

Sarah LUCIA-HOAGLAND and Julia PENELOPE (eds) (1988) *For Lesbians Only: A Separatist Anthology*, London: Onlywomen Press.

Lee LYNCH (1992) 'Cruising the libraries', in Karla JAY and Joanne GLASGOW (eds) *Lesbian Texts and Contexts: Radical Revisions*, London: Onlywomen Press.

Cynthia MACADAMS (1977) *Emergence*, New York: Chelsea House.

—— (1983) *Rising Goddess*, New York: Morgan and Morgan.

Susan McCLARY (1991) *Feminine Endings: Music, Gender and Sexuality*, University of Minnesota Press.

Lyndall MACCOWAN (1992) 'Recollecting history, renaming lives: femme stigma and the feminist seventies and eighties', in Joan NESTLE (ed.) *The Persistent Desire: A Femme/Butch Reader*, Boston: Alyson.

Christian McEWAN (ed.) (1988) *Naming the Waves: Contemporary Lesbian Poetry*, London: Virago.

Midge MACKENZIE (1975/1988) *Shoulder to Shoulder*, New York: Vintage Books.

Mary McINTOSH (1968) 'The homosexual role', in Kenneth PLUMMER (ed.) (1981) *The Making of the Modern Homosexual*, London: Hutchinson.

Jay McCLAREN (1992) *An Encyclopaedia of Gay and Lesbian Recordings*, (limited edition chapbook), Amsterdam.

Mavis MACLEAN and Dulcie GROVES (eds) *Women's Issues in Social Policy*, London: Routledge.

MADONNA (1992) *Sex*, New York: Times Warner.

Pat MAHONY (1983) 'Boys will be boys: teaching Women's Studies in mixed-sex groups', in *Women's Studies International Forum* 6(3).

—— (1989) 'Sexual violence and mixed schools', in Carol JONES and Pat MAHONY (eds) *Learning Our Lines: Sexuality and Social Control in Education*, London: The Women's Press.

Rosemary MANNING (1987) *A Corridor of Mirrors*, London: The Women's Press.

Del MARTIN and Phyllis LYON (1972) *Lesbian/Woman*, San Francisco: Bantam Books.

Jeffrey MASSON (1990) *Against Therapy*, London: Fortuna.

—— (1992) *The Assault on Truth: Freud and Child Sexual Abuse*, London: Fontana.

William MASTERS and Virginia JOHNSON (1979) *Homosexuality in Perspective*, Boston: Little, Brown and Co.

Elizabeth MEESE (1992) 'Theorising lesbian: writing – a love letter', in Karla JAY and Joanne GLASGOW (eds) *Lesbian Texts and Contexts: Radical Revisions*, London: Onlywomen Press.

Philip A. MELLOR and Chris SHILLING (1993) 'Modernity, self-identity and the sequestration of death', *Sociology* 27(3) August.

Jayne MELVILLE (n.d.) 'Lesbians in Entertainment' *Square Peg* 18: 18–19.

Kobena MERCER (1991) 'Skin head sex thing: racial difference and the homo-erotic imaginary', in BAD OBJECT-CHOICES (eds) *How Do I Look? Queer Film and Video*, Seattle: Bay Press.

Margaret MIES (1983) 'Towards a methodology of feminist research', in Gloria BOWLES and Renate DUELLI KLEIN (eds) *Theories of Women's Studies*, London: Routledge and Kegan Paul.

Agne MILES (1991) *Women, Health and Medicine*, Milton Keynes: Open University Press.

Kate MILLET (1970) *Sexual Politics*, London: Virago.

Jane MILLS (1989) *Womanwords*, London: Virago.

Juliet MITCHELL and Ann OAKLEY (eds) (1976) *The Rights and Wrongs of Women*, Harmondsworth: Penguin.

Tania MODLESKI (1991) *Feminism Without Women: Culture and Criticism in a 'Postfeminist' Age*, London: Routledge.

Robin MORGAN (ed.) (1984) *Sisterhood is Global: The International Women's Movement Anthology*, Harmondsworth: Penguin.

Martin MORIARTY (1993) 'Gays get raw deal on pension funds', *Public Service* (NALGO journal) February.

Frank MORT (1987) *Dangerous Sexualities: Medico-Moral Politics in England Since 1830*, London: Routledge and Kegan Paul.

Laura MULVEY (1972) 'Fears, fantasies and the male unconscious or "You don't know what is happening, do you Mr Jones?"' in *Visual and Other Pleasures*, London: Macmillan.

—— (1989) *Visual and Other Pleasures*, London: Macmillan.

Sally MUNT (ed.) (1992) *New Lesbian Criticism: Literary and Cultural Readings*, Hemel Hempstead: Harvester Wheatsheaf.

Suniti NAMJOSHI and Gillian HANSCOMBE (1986) *Flesh and Paper*, Seaton, Jezebel Books.

NATIONAL LESBIAN AND GAY SURVEY (1992) *What a Lesbian Looks Like: Writings by Lesbians on Their Lives and Lifestyles*, London: Routledge.

Suzanne NEILD and Roslind PEARSON (1992) *Women Like Us*, London: The Women's Press.

Gilles NERET (1992) *Tamara de Lempicka*, Koln: Benedikt Taschen Verlag.

Joan NESTLE (1987) *A Restricted Country*, London: Sheba.

—— (1992) 'Flamboyance and fortitude – an introduction', in *The Persistent Desire: A Femme/Butch Reader*, Boston: Alyson.

Julia NEUBERGER (1991) *Whatever's Happening to Women? Promises, Practices and Payoffs*, London: Kyle Cathie.

Angela NEUSTATTER (1989) *Hyenas in Petticoats: A Look at Twenty Years of Feminism*, London: Harrap.

NEW INTERNATIONALIST (eds) (1985) *Women: A World Report*, London: Methuen.

Fred NEWMAN (1992) *The Myth of Psychology*, New York: Castillo.

Vivien N.G. (1989) 'Homosexuality and the state in late imperial China', in DUBERMAN *et al.* (eds) (1991) *Hidden From History: Reclaiming the Gay and Lesbian Past*, Harmondsworth: Penguin.

Doris NIELD CHEW (1982) *Ada Nield Chew: The Life and Writings of a Working Woman*, London: Virago.

Linda NOCHLIN (1989) *Women, Art and Power and Other Essays*, London: Thames and Hudson.

William NORRIS (1992) 'Liberal attitudes and homophobic acts: the paradoxes of homosexual experience in a liberal institution', in Karen HARBECK (ed.) *Coming Out of the Classroom Closet*, New York: Harrington Park Press.

Rictor NORTON (1992) *Mother Clap's Molly House: the Gay Subculture in England, 1700–1830*, London, Gay Men's Press.

Ann OAKLEY (1976) 'Wisewoman and medicine man: changes in the management of childbirth', in Juliet MITCHELL and Ann OAKLEY (eds) *The Rights and Wrongs of Women*, Harmondsworth: Penguin.

—— (1980) *Woman Confined*, Harmondsworth: Penguin.

Mary O'BRIEN (1981) *The Politics of Reproduction*, London: Routledge and Kegan Paul.

Mary O'DONNELL, Kater POLLACK, Val LEOFFLER and Ziesel SAUNDERS (1979) *Lesbian Health Matters*, Santa Cruz Women's Health Collective.

ONLYWOMEN PRESS (ed.) (1981) *Love Your Enemy? The Debate Between Political Lesbianism and Heterosexual Feminism*, London: Onlywomen Press.

Susie ORBACH and Louise EICHENBAUM (1983) *What do Women Want?*, Glasgow: Fontana/Collins.

Rebecca O'ROURKE (1989) *Reflecting on 'The Well of Loneliness'*, London: Routledge.

Patrick ORR (1985) 'Sex bias in schools: national perspectives', in Judith WHYTE, Rosemary DEEM, Rosley KANT and Maureen CRUICKSHANK, (eds) *Girl Friendly Schooling*, London: Methuen.

Claire PAJACZKOWSKA (1992) 'The heterosexual presumption', in John CAUGHIE, Annete KUHN and Mandy MERCK (eds) *The Sexual Subject: A 'Screen' Reader in Sexuality*, London: Routledge.

Alice PARKER (1992) 'Nicole Brossard: a differential equation of lesbian love', in JAY and GLASGOW (eds) *Lesbian Texts and Contexts: Radical Revisions*, London: Onlywomen Press.

Pat PARKER (1978) *Movement in Black*, New York: Firebrand Books.

Roszika PARKER and Griselda POLLOCK (1981) *Old Mistresses: Women, Art and Ideology*, London: Routledge and Kegan Paul.

Gillian PASCAL (1986) *Social Policy: A Feminist Analysis*, London: Tavistock.

Carole PATEMAN (1992) 'Equality, difference and subordination: the politics of motherhood and women's citizenship', in Gisela BOCK and Susan JAMES (eds) *Beyond Equality and Difference: Citizenship, Feminist Politics and Female Subjectivity*, London: Routledge.

Cindy PATTON (1985) *Sex and Germs: The Politics of AIDS*, Boston: South End Press.

—— (1991) 'Unmediated lust? The improbable space of lesbian desires', in Tessa BOFFIN and Jean FRASER (eds) *Stolen Glances: Lesbians Take Photographs*, London: Pandora.

Julia PENELOPE and Sarah VALENTINE (eds) (1990) *Finding the Lesbians: Personal Accounts from Around the World*, Freedom: The Crossing Press.

Karen PETERSEN and J.J. WILSON (1976) *Women Artists: Recognition and Reappraisal from the Early Middle Ages to the Twentieth Century*, London: The Women's Press.

Suzanne PHARR (1988) *Homophobia: A Weapon of Sexism*, Little Rock, Arkansas: Chardon Press.

Charles PHILLIPS (1987) *Passion by Design: The Art and Times of Tamara de Lempicka*, Oxford: Phaidon.

PHOTOGRAPHERS AND FRIENDS UNITED AGAINST AIDS (1990) *The Indomitable Spirit* (exhibition catalogue), New York: Harry Abrams.

THE PINK BOOK EDITING TEAM (1988) *The Second ILGA Pink Book: A Global View of Lesbian and Gay Liberation and Oppression*, Rijksuniversiteit, Utrecht, Interfacultaire Werkgroep Homostudies.

Laura PITTER and Alexandra STIGLMAYER (1993) 'Bosnia: will the world remember? Can the women forget?' *Ms.* III(5) March/April.

Kenneth PLUMMER (1981a) 'Homosexual categories: some research problems in the labelling perspective of homosexuality', in PLUMMER (ed.) *The Making of the Modern Homosexual*, London: Hutchinson.

—— (1981b) 'Researching into homosexualities', in PLUMMER (ed.) *The Making of the Modern Homosexual*, London: Hutchinson.

—— (1992) 'Speaking its name: inventing a lesbian and gay studies', in PLUMMER (ed.) *Modern Homosexualities: Fragments of Lesbian and Gay Experience*, London: Routledge.

Melvin POHL (1988) 'Recovery from alcoholism and chemical dependency for lesbians and gay men', in Michael SHERNOFF and William STOTT (eds) *The Sourcebook of Lesbian/Gay Healthcare*, Washington: National Lesbian and Gay Health Foundation.

Griselda POLLOCK (1988) 'Screening the seventies: sexuality and representation', in *Vision and Difference: Femininity, Feminism and the History of Art*, London: Routledge.

Elena PONIATOWSKA and Carla STELLWEG (1992) *Frida Kahlo*, London: Chatto and Windus.

Barbara PONSE (1978) *Identities in the Lesbian World: The Social Construction of Self*, Westport: Greenwood Press.

Karl POPPER (1962) *Conjectures and Refutations*, London: Routledge and Kegan Paul.

Kevin PORTER and Jeffrey WEEKS (eds) (1991) *Between the Acts: Lives of Homosexual Men 1885–1967*, London: Routledge.

Quim 1–4 (Summer 1989, Summer 1991, Winters 1991 and 1992), London.

Jill RADFORD (1991) 'Immaculate conceptions', *Trouble and Strife* 21 (Summer).

RADICALESBIANS (1970) 'The woman-identified woman', in HOAGLAND and PENELOPE (eds) *For Lesbians Only: A Separatist Anthology*, London: Onlywomen Press.

Louise RAFKIN (ed.) (1990) *Different Mothers: Sons and Daughters of Lesbians Talk About their Lives*, Pittsburgh: Cleis Press.

Caroline RAMAZANOGLU (1989) *Feminism and the Contradictions of Oppression*, London: Routledge.

Nina RAPI (1990) 'Lesbian theatre', *Rouge* 5 (Winter).

—— (1991) 'Theatre of moments' *Rouge* 6 (April–June).

Adrienne RICH (1981a) 'Compulsory heterosexuality and lesbian existence', in (1987) *Blood, Bread and Poetry*, London: Virago.

—— (1981b) 'Disobedience and Women's Studies', in *Blood, Bread and Poetry*, London: Virago.

Dell RICHARDS (1990) *Lesbian Lists: A Look at Lesbian Culture, History and Personalities*, Boston: Alyson Press.

Diane RICHARDSON (1981) 'Lesbian identities', in John HART and Diane RICHARDSON (eds) *The Theory and Practice of Homosexuality*, London: Routledge and Kegan Paul.

—— (ed.) (1995) *Telling It Straight: Theorising Heterosexuality*, London: Open University Press.

RIGHTS OF WOMEN LESBIAN CUSTODY GROUP (1986) *Lesbian Mothers' Legal Handbook*, London: The Women's Press.

Tom ROBINSON with Andy SHEPHERD (1989) 'A conversation about rock, politics and gays', in Simon SHEPHERD and Mick WALLIS (eds) *Coming on Strong: Gay Politics and Culture*, London: Unwin Hyman.

Sarah ROELOFS (1991) 'Labour and the natural order: intentionally promoting heterosexuality', in KAUFMANN *et al.* (eds) *High Risk Lives: Lesbian and Gay Politics after THE CLAUSE*, Bridport, Prism Press.

Judith ROOF (1991) *A Lure of Knowledge: Lesbian Sexuality and Theory*, Columbia University Press.

Karen ROSS (1992) 'All facing a health crisis', in *The Pink Paper* 249, 25 October.

Sheila ROWBOTHAM (1973) *Hidden from History: Three Hundred Years of Women's Oppression and the Fight Against it*, London: Pluto Press.

ROYAL COLLEGE OF NURSING (ed.) (1992) *Health of Half the Nation*, London: Royal College of Nursing.

Gayle RUBIN (1984) 'Thinking sex: notes for a radical theory of the politics of sexuality', in Carol VANCE (ed.) *Pleasure and Danger: Exploring Female Sexuality*, London: Pandora.

Sonja RUEHL (1982) 'Inverts and experts: Radclyffe Hall and the lesbian identity', in Rosalnin BRUNT and Caroline ROWAN, *Feminism, Culture and Politics*, London: Lawrence and Wishart.

Hendrick RUITENBACK (ed.) (1963) *The Problem of Homosexuality in Modern Society*, New York: Dutton.

Jane RULE (1975) *Lesbian Images*, Freedom: The Crossing Press.

Leila J. RUPP (1989) '"Imagine my surprise": women's relationships in mid twentieth-century America', in DUBERMAN *et al.* (eds) *Hidden from History: Reclaiming the Gay and Lesbian Past*, Harmondsworth: Penguin.

Michael RUSE (1988) *Homosexuality: A Philosophical Enquiry*, Oxford: Basil Blackwell.

Barbara RUSKIN and Irene PADAVIC (1988) 'Supervisors as gatekeepers: male supervisors' response to women's integration in plant jobs', in *Social Problems* 35(5) (December).

Joanna RUSS (1983) *How to Suppress Women's Writing*, Austin: University of Texas.

Vito RUSSO (1981) *The Celluloid Closet*, New York: Harper and Row.

Jonathan RUTHERFORD (ed.) (1990) *Identity: Community, Culture, Difference*, London: Lawrence and Wishart.

Caitlin RYAN and Judith BRADFORD (1988) 'The national lesbian healthcare survey: an overview', in Michael SHERNOFF and William SCOTT (eds) *The Sourcebook on Lesbian/Gay Healthcare*, Washington: National Lesbian and Gay Health Foundation.

Gita SAHGAL and Nira YUVAL-DAVIS (eds) (1992) *Refusing Holy Orders: Women and Fundamentalism in Britain*, London: Virago.

SAMOIS (eds) (1981) *Coming to Power: Writings and Graphics on Lesbian S/M*, Boston: Alyson.

James SASLOW (1978) 'Closets in the museum: homophobia and art history', in Karla JAY and Allen YOUNG (eds) *Lavender Culture*, New York: Jove/HBJ.

Jan SCHIPPERS (1989) 'Homosexual identity: essentialism and constructionism', in Dennis ALTMAN *et al.*, *Which Homosexuality?*, London: Gay Men's Press.

Beth SCHNEIDER (1984) 'Peril and promise: lesbians workplace participation', in DARTY and POTTER (eds) *Women-Identified Women*, Paolo Alto: Mayfield.

—— (1992) 'Lesbian politics and AIDS work', in PLUMMER (ed.) *Modern Homosexualities: Fragments of Lesbian and Gay Experience*, London: Routledge.

Percy SCHOLES (1969) *The Oxford Companion to Music*, Oxford: Oxford University Press.

Cathy SCHWICHTENBERG (ed.) (1993) *The Madonna Connection: Representational Politics, Subcultural Identities and Cultural Theory*, San Francisco: Westview Press.

Marion SCOTT (1980) 'Teach her a lesson: sexist curriculum in patriarchal education', in Dale SPENDER and Elizabeth SARAH (eds) *Learning to Lose: Sexism and Education*, London: The Women's Press.

Sara SCOTT (1983) 'Holding on to what we've won', *Trouble and Strife* 1 (Winter).

Roger SCRUTON (1986) *Sexual Desire*, London: Weidenfeld and Nicolson.

Jonis SEAGER and Ann OLSON (1986) *Women in the World: An International Atlas*, London: Pan Books.

James T. SEARS (1991) *Growing Up Gay in the South: Race, Gender and Journeys of the Spirit*, New York: The Haworth Press.

Eve Kosofksy SEDGWICK (1985) *Between Men: English Literature and Male Homosocial Desire*, New York: Columbia University Press.

—— (1991) *Epistemology of the Closet*, London: Harvester Wheatsheaf.

Lynne SEGAL (1994) *Straight Sex: The Politics of Pleasure*, London: Virago.

Lynne SHAPIRO (1978) 'The growing business behind women's music', in JAY and YOUNG (eds) *Laveder Culture*, New York: Jove/HBJ.

Simon SHEPHERD (1989) 'Gay sex spy orgy: the state's need for queers', in SHEPHERD and WALLIS (eds) *Coming on Strong: Gay Politics and Culture*, London: Unwin Hyman.

Simon SHEPHERD and Mick WALLIS (eds) (1989) *Coming on Strong: Gay Politics and Culture*, London: Unwin Hyman.

Susan SHERIDAN (1991) 'From margin to mainstream: situating women's studies', in Sneja GUNEW (ed.) *A Reader in Feminist Knowledge*, London: Routledge.

Elaine SHOWALTER (1985) *The Female Malady: Women, Madness and English Culture 1830–1980*, London: Virago.

Charles SILVERSTEIN (1991) 'Psychological and medical treatments of homosexuality', in John C. GONSIOREK and James D. WEINRICH (eds) *Homosexuality: Research Implications for Public Policy*, London: Sage.

Carol SMART (ed.) (1992) *Regulating Womanhood: Historical Essays on Marriage, Motherhood and Sexuality*, London: Routledge.

Cherry SMYTH (1990) 'The pleasure threshold: looking at lesbian pornography on film', *Feminist Review* 34, Spring: 'Perverse politics: the lesbian issue'.

—— (1992) *Lesbians Talk Queer Notions*, London: Scarlet Press.

Ethyl SMYTH (abridged/edited by Ronald CRICHTON) (1990) *The Memoirs of Ethyl Smyth*, London: Viking.

Anne SNITOW, Chrissie STANSELL and Sharon THOMPSON (1984) *Desire: The Politics of Sexuality*, London: Virago.

Susan SONTAG (1977) *On Photography*, Harmondsworth: Penguin.

Diana SOUHAMI (1988) *Gluck: Her Biography*, London: Pandora.

—— (1991) *Gertrude and Alice*, London: Pandora.

Dale SPENDER (1982) *Women of Ideas and What Men have Done to Them: Aphra Behn to Adrienne Rich*, London: Routledge and Kegan Paul.

—— (1985: 2nd ed.) *Man-Made Language*, London: Routledge and Kegan Paul.

—— (1986) *Mothers of the Novel*, London: Pandora.

Lynne SPENDER (1983) *Intruders on the Rights of Men: Women's Unpublished Heritage*, London: Pandora.

Robert STAM, Robert BURGOYNE and Sandy FLITTERMAN-LEWIS (1992) *New Vocabularies in Film Semiotics: Structuralism, Post-Structuralism and Beyond*, London: Routledge.

Liz STANLEY (1990) 'Feminist praxis and the academic mode of production: an editorial introduction' in *Feminist Praxis: Research, Theory and Epistemology in Feminist Sociology*, London: Routledge.

—— (1992) 'Epistemological issues in researching lesbian history', in Hilary

HINDS, Ann PHOENIX and Jackie STACEY (eds) *Working Out: New Directions for Women's Studies*, London: Falmer.

Liz STANLEY and Sue WISE (1979) 'Feminist consciousness, feminist research and experiences of sexism', *Women Studies International Quarterly* 2: 359–74.

Michelle STANWORTH (1987) 'Girls on the margins: a study of gender divisions in the classroom', in Gaby WEINER and Madeleine ARNOT (eds) *Gender under Scrutiny*, Milton Keynes: Open University Press.

Gertrude STEIN (1933) *The Autobiography of Alice B. Toklas*, Harmondsworth: Penguin.

Stephen STEWART (1985) *Positive Image: A Portrait of Gay America*, New York: William Morrow and Co.

Catharine R. STIMPSON (1981) 'Zero degree deviancy: the lesbian novel in English', in STIMPSON (ed.) (1985) *Where the Meanings Are: Feminism and Cultural Spaces*, London: Routledge.

—— (1992) 'Afterword: lesbian studies in the 1990s', in JAY and GLASGOW (eds) *Lesbian Texts and Contexts: Radical Revisions*, London: Onlywomen Press.

Ann STOKES (1985) *A Studio of One's Own*, Tallahassee: Naiad Press.

Anthony STORR (1964) *Sexual Deviation*, Harmondsworth: Penguin.

Elizabeth STUART (1992) *Daring to Speak Love's Name: A Gay and Lesbian Prayer Book*, London: Hamish Hamilton.

Maud SULTER (ed.) (1990) *Passion: Discourses on Blackwomen's Creativity*, Hebden Bridge: Urban Fox Press.

John Addington SYMONDS (1928; reprinted 1984) *Sexual Inversion*, New York: Bell.

Thomas SZASZ (1962) *The Myth of Mental Illness*, St Albans: Paladin.

—— (1974) *The Manufacture of Madness*, St Albans: Paladin.

Donna TANNER (1978) *The Lesbian Couple*, Toronto: Lexington Books.

Beverly THIELE (1992) 'Vanishing acts in social and political thought: tricks of the trade', in Linda MCDOWELL and Rosemary PRINGLE (eds) *Defining Women: Social Institutions and Gender Divisions*, Cambridge: Polity Press.

Philip THOMAS (1991) 'Girls just wanna have fun', *Empire*, August.

Lisa TICKNER (1987) 'The body politic: female sexuality and women artists since 1970', in Rosemary BETTERTON (ed.) *Looking On: Images of Femininity in the Visual Arts and Media*, London: Pandora.

TIME (no credit) (1970) 'Women's lib: a second look', *Time*, 14 December: 50.

Rosemarie TONG (1989) *Feminist Thought: A Comprehensive Introduction*, London: Routledge.

Evelyn TORTON-BECK (1982) *Nice Jewish Girls: A Lesbian Anthology*, Trumansburg: The Crossing Press.

Peter TOWNSEND, Neil DAVIDSON and Margaret WHITEHEAD (eds) (1987) *Inequaliies in Health: the Black Report and the Health Divide*, Harmondsworth: Penguin.

Valerie TRAUB (1991) 'The ambiguities of "Lesbian viewing pleasure": the (dis)articulations of "Black Widow"', in Julia EPSTEIN and Kristina STRAUB (eds) *Body Guards: The Cultural Politics of Gender Ambiguity*, London: Routledge.

Lorraine TRENCHARD (ed.) (1984) *Talking about Young Lesbians*, London Gay Teenage Group.

—— (1989) *Being Lesbian*, London: Gay Men's Press.

Lorraine TRENCHARD and Hugh WARREN (1984) 'Talking about school: the experiences of young lesbians and gay men', in WEINER and ARNOT (eds) *Gender under Scrutiny*, Milton Keynes: Open University Press.

Jane USSHER (1991) *Women's Madness: Misogyny or Mental Illness?*, London: Harvester Wheatsheaf.

Alison UTTLEY (1993) 'When hetero becomes another dirty word', *The Times Higher Education Supplement* 26 February.

Carol VANCE (ed.) (1984) *Pleasure and Danger: Exploring Female Sexuality*, London: Pandora.

—— (1989) 'Social construction theory: problems in the history of sexuality', in Dennis ALTMAN *et al.*, *Homosexuality, Which Homosexuality?*, London: Gay Men's Press.

Ethlie Ann VARE and Greg PTACEK (1987) *Mothers of Invention: From the Bra to the Bomb, Forgotten Women and Their Unforgettable Ideas*, New York: William Morrow.

Martha VICINUS (1989) '"They wonder to which sex I belong": the historical roots of the modern lesbian identity', in Dennis ALTMAN *et al.*, *Homosexuality, Which Homosexuality?*, London: Gay Men's Press.

Ginny VIDA (ed.) (1978) *Our Right to Love: A Lesbian Resource Book*, Englewood Cliffs: Prentice Hall.

Alice WALKER (1981) *In Search of Our Mothers' Gardens*, London: Women's Press.

Valerie WALKERDINE (1987) 'Sex power and pedagogy', in Madeline ARNOT and Gaby WEINER (eds) *Gender and the Politics of Schooling*, London: Hutchinson/Open University.

Cellestine WARE (1970) *Woman Power: The Movement for Women's Liberation*, New York: Tower.

Vron WARE (1992) *Beyond the Pale: White Women, Racism and History*, London: Verso.

Betsy WARLAND (ed.) (1991) *Inversions: Writings by Dykes, Queers and Lesbians*, London: Open Letters.

Simon WATNEY (1987) *Policing Desire: Pornography, AIDS and the Media*, London: Commedia.

—— (1992) 'My kid brother is sick', *The Pink Paper* 250, 1 November.

Christine WEBB (1993) 'The health of single, never-married women in old age', *Journal of Advances in Health and Nursing Care* 1(6).

Wendy WEBSTER (1992) 'Our life: working-class women's autobiography in Britain', in Frances BONNER, *Lizbeth GOODMAN, Richard ALLEN, Linda JAMES and Catherine KING (eds) Imagining Women: Cultural Representations and Gender*, Cambridge: Polity Press.

Chris WEEDON (1987) *Feminist Practice and Poststructuralist Theory*, Oxford: Basil Blackwell.

Jeffrey WEEKS (1977, 1990) *Coming Out: Homosexual Politics in Britain from the Nineteenth Century to the Present*, London: Quartet.

—— (1985) *Sexuality and Its Discontents*, London: Routledge and Kegan Paul.

—— (1986) *Sexuality*, London: Routledge.

—— (1987) 'Questions of identity' in Pat CAPLAN (ed.) *The Cultural Construction of Sexuality*, London: Routledge.

Marsha WEIDNER, Allen JOHNSTON LAING, Irving YUCHENG LO, Christine CHU and James ROBINSON (1988) *Views from Jade Terrace: Chinese Women Artists 1300–1912*, Indianapolis Museum of Art and Rizzoli, New York.

Gaby WEINER and Madeleine ARNOT (eds) (1987) *Gender under Scrutiny*, Milton Keynes: Open University Press.

James WEINRICH (1990) 'Reality or Social Contruction?', in Edward STEIN (ed.) *Forms of Desire: Sexual Orientation and the Social Constructions Controversy*, London: Routledge.

James D. WEINRICH and Walter L. WILLIAMS (1991) 'Strange customs, familiar lives: homosexualities in other cultures', in John GONSIOREK and James WEINRICH (eds) *Homosexuality: Research Implications for Public Policy*, London: Sage.

Andrea WEISS (1992) *Vampires and Violets: Lesbians in the Cinema*, London: Jonathan Cape.

Jess WELLS (1982) *A Herstory of Prositution in Western Europe*, Berkeley, Shameless Hussy Press.

Chris WHITE (1992) '"Poets and Lovers Evermore": the poetry and journals of Michael Field', in Joseph BRISTOW (ed.) *Sexual Sameness: Textual Differences in Lesbian and Gay Writing*, London: Routledge.

Patricia WHITE (1991) 'Female spectator, lesbian specter: "The Haunting"', in Diana FUSS (ed.) *Inside/Out: Lesbian Theories, Gay Theories*, London: Routledge.

Harriet WHITEHEAD (1981) 'The bow and the burden strap: a new look at institutionalized homosexuality in Native North America', in Sherry ORTNER and Harriet WHITEHEAD (eds) *Sexual Meanings: The Cultural Construction of Gender and Sexuality*, Cambridge University Press.

Cheyl WIESENFELD, Yvonne KALMUS, Sonia KATCHIAN and Rikki RIPP (eds) (1976) *Women See Women*, New York: Thomas Y. Crowell Co.

Sue WILKINSON and Celia KITZINGER (1993) 'Theorizing heterosexuality: editorial introduction', in *Heterosexuality: A Feminism and Psychology Reader*, London: Sage.

Jenny WILLIAMS (1987) 'The construction of women and black students as educational problems: re-evaluating policy on gender and race', in ARNOT and WEINER (eds) *Gender and the Politics of Schooling*, London: Hutchinson/Open University.

Linda WILLIAMS (1990) *Hard Core*, London: Pandora.

Val WILLIAMS (1986) *Women Photographers: The Other Observers: 1900 to the Present*, London: Virago.

Amrit WILSON (1978) *Finding a Voice: Asian Women in Britain*, London: Virago.

Anna WILSON (1992) 'Lorde and the African–American tradition' in Sally MUNT (ed.) *New Lesbian Criticism*, London: Harvester Wheatsheaf.

Elizabeth WILSON (1992) 'Feminist fundamentalism: the shifting politics of sex and censorship', in Lynne SEGAL and Mary McINTOSH (eds) *Sex Exposed: Sexuality and the Pornography Debate*, London: Virago.

Tamsin WILTON (1992a) *Antibody Politic: AIDS and Society*, Cheltenham: New Clarion Press.

—— (1992b) 'Desire and the politics of representation: issues for lesbians and heterosexual women', in Hilary HINDS, Ann PHOENIX and Jackie STACEY (eds) *Working Out: New Directions for Women's Studies*, London: Falmer Press.

—— (1993a) 'Queer subjects: lesbians, heterosexual women and the academy', in Mary KENNEDY, Cathy LUBELSKA and Val WALSH (eds) *Making Connections: Women's Studies, Women's Movements, Women's Lives*, London: Taylor and Francis.

—— (1993b) 'Sisterhood in the service of patriarchy: heterosexual women's friendships and male power', in Sue WILKINSON and Celia KITZINGER (eds) *Heterosexuality: A Feminism and Psychology Reader*, London: Sage.

—— (1994a) 'The "L" Word: an exploration of the meanings of the word "lesbian"' (unpublished paper).

—— (1994b) 'Feminism and the erotics of health promotion', in Lesley DOYAL, Jennie NAIDOO and Tamsin WILTON (eds) *AIDS: Setting a Feminist Agenda*, London: Falmer Press.

—— (1995) *Immortal, Invisible: Lesbians, and the Moving Image*, London: Routledge.

—— (1995) 'Researching Lesbian Health', paper given at 'Researching Women, Gender and Health Conference', University of the West of England, June.

Mary WINGS (1992a) *Divine Victim*, London: The Women's Press.

—— (1992b) 'Rebecca: a lesbian re-reading', paper given at 'Activating theory: Lesbian and Gay studies Conference', York University, November.

Monique WITTIG (1975) *The Lesbian Body*, New York: William Morrow.

—— (1981) 'One is not born a woman', in Monique WITTIG (1992) *The Straight Mind and Other Essays*, London: Harvester Wheatsheaf.

Deborah Goleman WOLF (1979) *The Lesbian Community*, Berkeley: University of California Press.

James WOOD (1993) 'The good Freud guide', *Weekend Guardian*, 25/26 August.

Virginia WOOLF (1928) *Orlando*, London: Hogarth Press.

—— (1929) *A Room of One's Own*, Harmondsworth: Penguin.

—— (1938) *Three Guineas*, London: Hogarth Press.

Thomas YINGLING (1991) 'AIDS in America: postmodern governance, identity and experience', in Diana FUSS (ed.) *Inside/Out: Lesbian Theories, Gay Theories*, London: Routledge.

Bonnie ZIMMERMAN (1985) 'What has never been: an overview of lesbian feminist literary criticism', in Elaine SHOWALTER (ed.) *The New Feminist Criticism*, London: Virago.

—— (1992a) *The Safe Sea of Women: Lesbian Fiction 1969–1989*, London: Onlywomen Press.

—— (1992b) 'Lesbians like this and like that: some notes on lesbian criticism for the nineties', in Sally MUNT (ed.) *New Lesbian Criticism: Literary and Cultural Readings*, London: Harvester Wheatsheaf.

Index